# A synopsis of
# RENAL DISEASES

**A. M. DAVISON**

**BSc MD FRCP**

*Consultant Renal Physician*
*St James's University Hospital, Leeds*

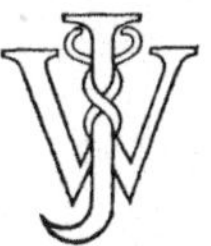

**BRISTOL**
**JOHN WRIGHT & SONS LTD**

Published by John Wright & Sons Ltd, 42–44 Triangle West, Bristol, BS8 1EX.


*British Library Cataloguing in Publication Data*
Davison, A. M.
    A synopsis of renal diseases.
    1. Kidneys – Diseases
    I. Title
    616.6'1    RC902


ISBN 0 7236 0569 6


Printed in Great Britain by Billing & Sons Ltd, Guildford, London and Worcester.

This book is written primarily for the undergraduate student and the postgraduate preparing for the MRCP examination. I hope it will also provide a quick ready reference to all interested in renal disease.

Nephrology has now 'come of age' and is a growing and exciting specialty. Because the kidneys are of prime importance in maintaining a stable internal environment there is no system free from involvement in the patient with renal disease. There is a tendency to consider nephrology as dialysis and transplantation and I hope that in this book I have dispelled this thought by describing the wide range of diseases affecting the kidney. In the past there has been considerable confusion regarding the terminology of renal diseases and in this volume I have tried to use the current generally accepted nomenclature.

I am very grateful to a number of colleagues for their helpful advice during the preparation of this text; in particular Professor G. R. Giles, Drs Hugo Mascie-Taylor, Vic Standing and David Thomson. The illustrations are the work of The Department of Medical Illustration, St James's University Hospital.

My thanks are due to Mr Roy Baker and Mr Adrian Symons of John Wright & Sons Ltd for their help and encouragement over the past year. I am indebted to Miss Gillian Best who typed the manuscripts with such enthusiasm. Finally I owe most to Marion, Andrew, Pamela and Iain for their support, encouragement and forbearance during the preparation of this book.

A.M.D.

# CONTENTS

# Chapter 1

# ANATOMY

Gross anatomy – Blood supply – Lymphatic drainage – Nerve supply – The nephron – The glomerulus – The juxtaglomerular complex – Embryology – Anatomical relations – The ureters – The bladder

## GROSS ANATOMY

The kidneys are paired structures which lie on the posterior abdominal wall behind the peritoneum. In the adult the bipolar length is approximately 13 cm but in view of the variation in body size a useful rule is that the bipolar length is approximately that of three lumbar vertebrae. In the child the size is relatively larger.

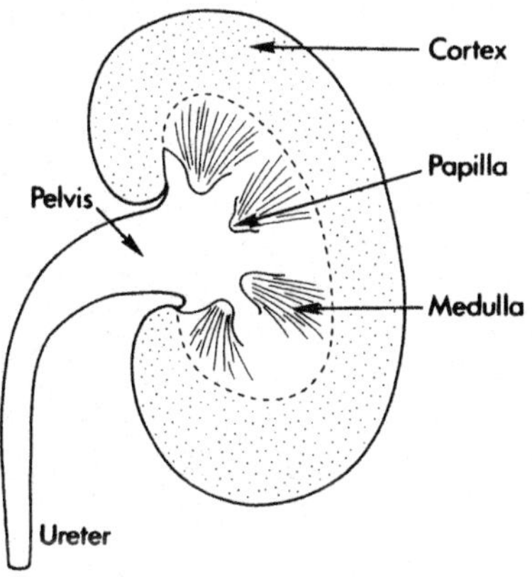


*Fig.* 1.1. Coronal section of kidney.

The external surfaces of the kidney are smooth and covered by a capsule. The lateral surface is convex and the medial surface is concave (the hilum). Through the hilum the renal artery, vein, nerves and the renal pelvis pass. If the kidney is bisected coronally two distinct parts may be identified (*Fig.* 1.1). The cortex has a granular appearance and is situated in the area immediately under the capsule. The medulla has a striate appearance which shows radiations from the tip of the papillae to the corticomedullary junction. This is due to the structure of the nephron with its glomerulus and convoluted tubules being in the cortex while the straight loop of Henle and collecting duct are situated in the medulla.

## BLOOD SUPPLY

The renal arteries arise from the aorta at the level of the second lumbar vertebra. The right artery passes posterior to the inferior vena cava. At the hilum the arteries divide into anterior and posterior divisions which in turn divide into interlobar arteries. These arteries then divide at the cortico-medullary junction and turn through a right angle to form the arcuate

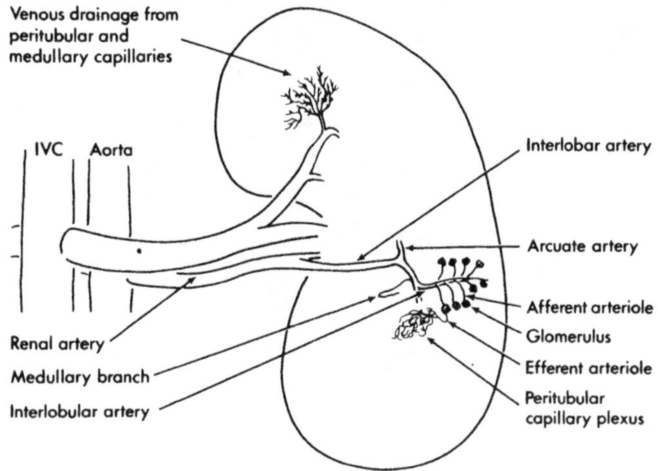


*Fig.* 1.2. Vascular supply of the kidney.

arteries, from which branches pass out into the cortex to form the inter-lobular arteries, while others branch into the medulla.

The interlobular arteries as they pass through the cortex give branches which form intralobular arteries. These vessels then divide into afferent arterioles which enter the glomeruli where they form a capillary plexus and then converge into an efferent arteriole which then forms a secondary capillary plexus around the tubules (*Fig.* 1.2).

The blood supply to the upper one-third to two-thirds of the ureter arises from the renal artery as it passes through the hilum.

There is considerable variation in arterial supply and multiple renal arteries are common (present in about one-third of normal people). Aberrant arteries to the lower pole are twice as common as those to the upper pole.

The venous drainage is essentially a mirror of the arterial supply.

## LYMPHATIC DRAINAGE

The lymphatic drainage follows the course of the renal arterial supply.

## NERVE SUPPLY

Sympathetic fibres arise from the spinal segments T11 and L1 and pass to the kidney by the coeliac and aortico-renal ganglia.

Parasympathetic fibres arise from the vagus and pelvic splanchnic nerves.

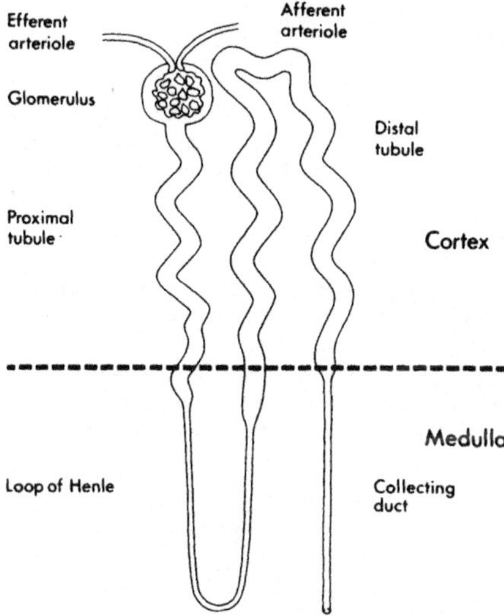


*Fig.* 1.3. Structure of the nephron.

## THE NEPHRON

Each kidney is composed of about one million nephrons. The nephron is the functional part of the kidney and is composed of the glomerulus, a proximal convoluted tubule, the loop of Henle, the distal convoluted tubule and the collecting tubule leading into the collecting duct (*Fig.* 1.3). The glomeruli and the convoluted tubules are situated in the cortex while the loop of Henle and collecting ducts are in the medulla. There is considerable heterogeneity in the structure of nephrons. The nephrons at the corticomedullary junction have long loops of Henle while those in the outer part of the cortex may have very short loops.

The tubular cells vary considerably in their structure along the nephron. In the proximal tubule the epithelium consists of low columnar cells containing many mitochondria. The luminal surface consists of a brush border of microvilli which project into the lumen while the basal surface is deeply indented. The descending limb of the loop of Henle has fairly thin and flat cells while soon after the tip of the loop the ascending limb consists of cuboidal cells. Similar cells are seen in the distal tubule which is shorter than the proximal. In the collecting duct the cells are of a low cuboid type.

## THE GLOMERULUS

The glomerulus is the functioning filtering unit of the nephron. It consists of a unique type of capillary plexus supported by a stalk known as the mesangium. As the afferent arteriole enters the glomerulus it divides into numerous capillary loops. These loops consist of finely fenestrated endothelial cells which sit on a basement membrane which has a homogeneous appearance and is composed of mucopolysaccharide. Surrounding the membrane are the epithelial cells which have numerous projections which interdigitate with adjacent cells. These projections are known as podocytes and they lie on the outer surface of the membrane (*Fig.* 1.4).

The stalk or supporting framework of the glomerular capillaries is the mesangium. This consists of a matrix which appears to offer continuity between the subendothelial space of the capillary wall through to the juxtaglomerular complex. The mesangium contains cells and in addition material which appears similar to the basement membrane.

Bowman's capsule consists of a layer of parietal epithelial cells which are squamous in type.

## THE JUXTAGLOMERULAR COMPLEX

The juxtaglomerular complex consists of the juxtaglomerular apparatus, the macula densa and the mesangium of the vascular pole of the glomerulus (*Fig.* 1.5).

The juxtaglomerular apparatus consists of highly granulated cells which are derived from the smooth muscle layer of the afferent arteriole. The granules are considered to be secretory granules and are probably a precursor of renin. Within the juxtaglomerular apparatus are also nerve fibres

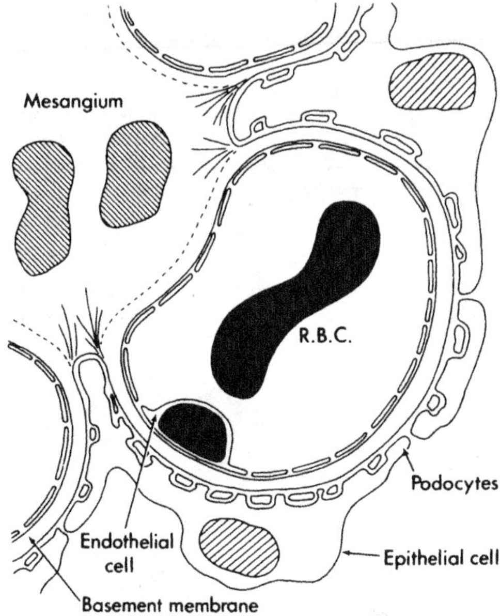


*Fig.* 1.4. Ultrastructure of the glomerulus.

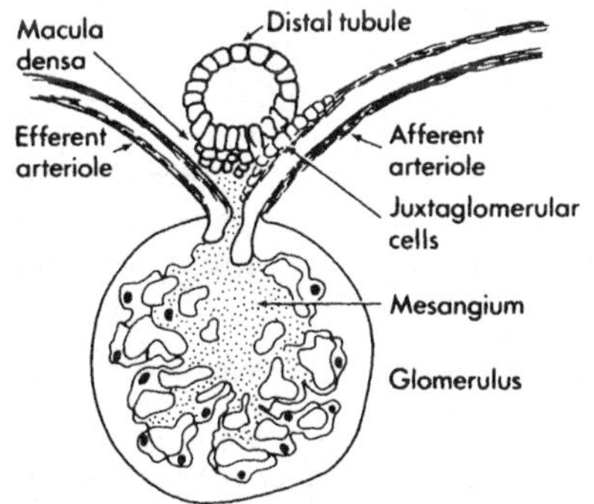


*Fig.* 1.5. Structure of the juxtaglomerular apparatus.

and ordinary arteriole smooth muscle cells which appear to contain micro-vesicles. A thin layer of endothelial cells separates the juxtaglomerular cells from the lumen of the afferent arteriole.

The macula densa is a specialised part of the distal tubule where it comes into close apposition to the vascular pole of the glomerulus. The distal tubule lies between the afferent arteriole, the efferent arteriole and the mesangium. The cells are similar to other distal tubular cells but they have projections which penetrate the mesangium.

## EMBRYOLOGY

Prior to the development of the permanent kidney from the metanephros two other structures arise and disappear in the embryo. All three structures

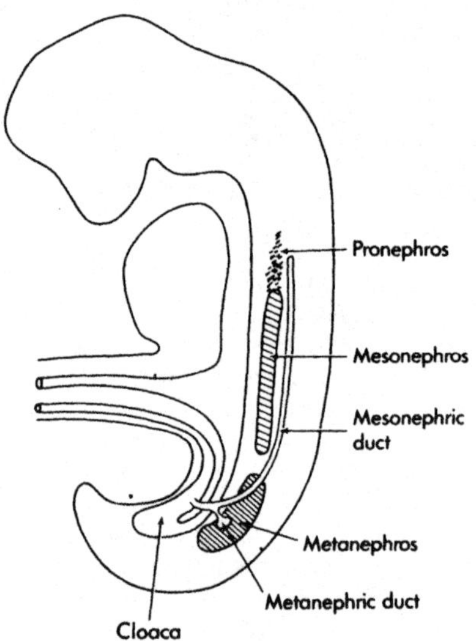


*Fig.* 1.6. Development of the kidney.

originate from the *nephrogenic cord* which develops from the intermediate mesoderm (*Fig.* 1.6).

The *pronephros* is found during the 4th and 5th weeks of development and arises in the cervical region. It is probably functionless.

The *mesonephros* is found from the 4th to about the 9th week. It extends from the upper thoracic to the lower lumbar segments. Tubules are formed and open into the *mesonephric duct*, which in turn opens into the cloaca. Branches from the abdominal aorta form primitive glomeruli. The tubules in their proximal part are lined by tall columnar epithelium and are probably functional in an excretory capacity. Degeneration of this system starts in the 5th week and proceeds caudally.

The *metanephros* forms the definitive kidney and develops from the mesonephric duct and from the caudal undifferentiated tissue of the nephrogenic cord which is termed the 'metanephrogenic cap'. From the mesonephric duct an outgrowth, the *ureteric bud*, develops and forms the ureter, pelvis and collecting tubules of the kidney. The metanephrogenic cap forms the rest of the kidney. Tubular function probably starts at about 10 weeks although formation of new nephrons continues until birth. At birth a number of nephrons are not fully differentiated and so function is not fully mature until shortly after. The kidney first develops in the pelvis and migrates upwards. The blood supply is originally obtained from the common iliac artery but during migration a series of vessels develop which involute once the renal artery is formed.

The bladder is formed from the cloaca by the development of a coronally arranged septum which splits the cloaca into two parts, the dorsal rectum and a ventral urogenital sinus from which the bladder is formed.

**Developmental Abnormalities**
KIDNEYS AND URETERS
1. Congenital cystic disease: due to failure of the union of the ureteric bud with the metanephrogenic cap or persistence of tubules which normally involute.
2. Horseshoe kidney: due to fusion of the two metanephric masses.
3. Pelvic kidney: from failure to ascend from the primary developmental position.
4. Double ureter: due to the formation of two ureteric buds. The ureter may fuse at any point in its length or both may enter the bladder separately.
5. Hypoplastic kidney: due to poor differentiation in the metanephros. May be unilateral or bilateral.
6. Aberrant renal artery: due to persistence of the early developmental arteries.
7. Absence: From failure of development of a metanephros on one side.
BLADDER
1. Persistent cloaca: failure of the urorectal septum.
2. Ectopia vesicae: failure of development of the infra-umbilical anterior wall.
3. Abnormal opening of the ureter into the urethra, seminal vesicle or vagina.
4. Abnormal opening of the urethra: hypospadias.

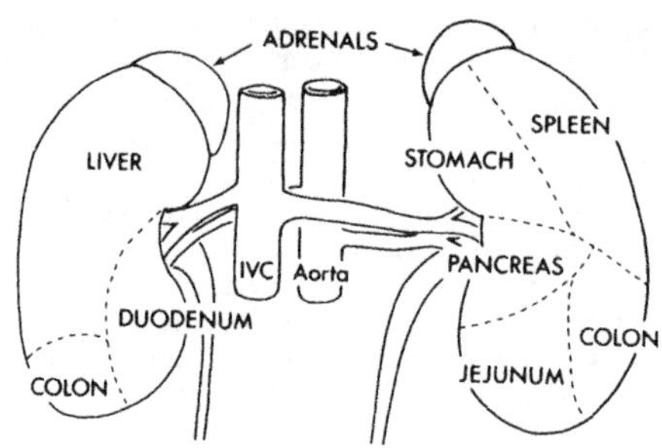


*Fig.* 1.7. Anterior relations of the kidney.

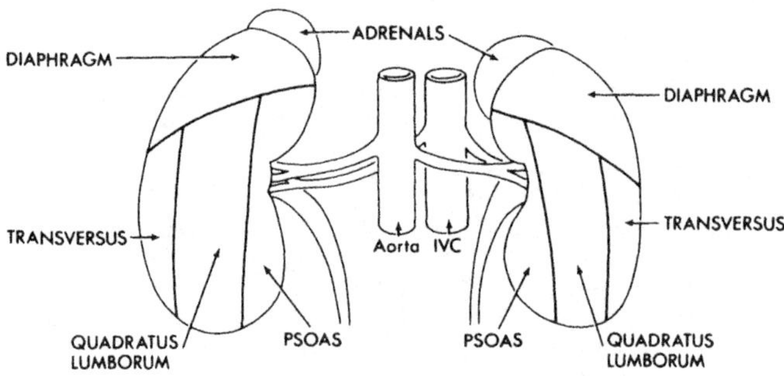


*Fig.* 1.8. Posterior relations of the kidney.

## ANATOMICAL RELATIONS

The anterior and posterior relations of the kidneys are shown in *Figs.* 1.7 and 1.8.

## THE URETERS

The collecting ducts of the nephrons open at the tip of the papillae and drain into the calyceal system. Normally there are six minor calyces in each kidney and these open into two or three major calyces which in turn join to form the renal pelvis, the enlarged upper end of the ureter.

The ureters are two muscular tubes which connect the renal pelvis to the bladder. The upper part of the ureter receives its blood supply from the renal artery while the middle and lower parts receive blood from lumbar vessels and the arteries of the bladder.

The ureters enter the bladder by passing obliquely through the muscular wall. This peculiar arrangement prevents urine passing up the ureter on bladder contraction and evacuation.

## THE BLADDER

The bladder is a hollow muscular organ which stores urine which is subsequently voided intermittently through the urethra.

The nerve supply to the bladder involves both autonomic and somatic nerves. The autonomic nerves consist of parasympathetic fibres of the pelvic splanchnic nerves from the 2nd, 3rd and 4th sacral segments and convey the sensation of the desire to micturate. The sympathetic nerves are from the hypogastric plexus but probably play little part in normal micturition. The pudendal nerve contains fibres from the 2nd, 3rd and 4th sacral nerves and provide efferent nerves to the external sphincter and afferent nerves from the posterior urethra.

Micturition is basically a spinal reflex which is facilitated and inhibited from higher centres. On micturition the perineal muscles and the external sphincter relax and the muscle of the bladder wall contracts.

# Chapter 2

# PHYSIOLOGY

Introduction – Renal blood flow – Autoregulation of renal blood flow – Glomerular filtration – Tubular function – Urine concentration and dilution – Sodium excretion – Potassium excretion – Chloride excretion – Urea excretion – Regulation of acid-base – Amino acid metabolism – Renin–angiotensin system – Erythropoietin – Antidiuretic hormone – Disorders of micturition

## INTRODUCTION

The kidneys are excretory organs but, in addition, they perform metabolic functions and have endocrine activity. The prime function is the maintenance of the internal environment by controlling the quality of the extracellular fluid. To achieve this a large volume of filtrate is formed which is modified as it passes along the nephron so that essential nutrients are retained, waste products are eliminated and water is conserved depending on the needs of the body. It is for this reason that the kidneys are extremely metabolically active requiring a high blood flow. The metabolic function includes the formation of certain amino acids and the detoxification of drugs. The endocrine activity is in the formation of renin and erythropoietin and the hydroxylation of cholecalciferol. A firm knowledge of the physiology of the kidney affords the best basis for understanding the consequences of disordered function.

## RENAL BLOOD FLOW

The blood flow to the kidneys is in the region of 1300 ml/min. This high flow rate accounts for 25 per cent of the cardiac output and produces a flow of approximately 4–5 ml/g/min. The distribution within the kidney is uneven with the cortex receiving five times as much blood per gram of tissue as the medulla.

The renal plasma flow can be measured by the Fick principle, i.e. by measuring the amount of a given substance taken up in unit time and dividing this value by the arteriovenous difference for the substance in the renal artery and renal vein. It is commonly measured by infusing para-aminohippuric acid (PAH) because of the high renal extraction by filtration and secretion. The value obtained by this method is an underestimate of the true renal plasma flow because a percentage of the blood entering the kidney is distributed to such non-excretory areas as the renal capsule. It does, however, provide an effective renal plasma flow and from the haematocrit the renal blood flow can be calculated.

The renal blood vessels are under the influence of vasoconstrictor sympathetic nerves and they also respond to adrenaline, noradrenaline and angiotensin. No vasodilator nerves have been demonstrated. Adrenaline and noradrenaline in small doses produce constriction of the efferent arterioles and so glomerular filtration is not significantly altered. Larger doses, however, produce constriction of both efferent and afferent arterioles with a subsequent diminution of filtration.

**Factors influencing Renal Plasma Flow**

| *Increase* | *Decrease* |
|---|---|
| Supine position | Upright posture |
| Pregnancy | Hypoxia |
| Pyrogens | Haemorrhage |
| High protein diet | Salt and water depletion |
| | Pain |
| | Vigorous exercise |
| | Emotion |

## AUTOREGULATION OF RENAL BLOOD FLOW

The renal blood flow is maintained fairly constant over a wide range of blood pressure. As the arterial mean pressure is increased to about 70 mmHg there is a direct increase in renal blood flow, but as the pressure is increased from 70 to 200 mmHg there is little increase in flow. The mechanism is probably mediated by a direct effect of the increased pressure on the smooth muscle of the afferent arteriole. By this means the glomerular filtration rate is maintained constant over a wide range of systemic blood pressure.

## GLOMERULAR FILTRATION

The production of urine begins with the formation of an ultrafiltrate of plasma by the glomerulus. This filtrate passes along the nephron and its composition is adjusted so that by the time it is discharged from the collecting duct into the pelvis of the kidney it has the composition of urine.

The ultrafiltrate of plasma is formed by the passage of fluid and solutes from the glomerular capillary lumen through the capillary wall and into Bowman's space. The filtrate is almost protein free but is iso-osmotic with respect to plasma and contains urea, creatinine, glucose and electrolytes in similar concentrations to those present in plasma. The force responsible for filtration is the hydrostatic pressure within the capillaries. This is opposed by the colloid osmotic pressure of the plasma and the pressure within Bowman's space. The effective filtration pressure is therefore:

capillary hydrostatic pressure — (colloid osmotic pressure +
Bowman's space hydrostatic pressure),

and amounts to approximately 25 mmHg.

The glomerular filtration rate remains remarkable constant over a wide range of blood pressure. This is achieved by the autoregulation of renal blood flow (*vide supra*) and by control of the tone of the afferent and efferent arterioles to compensate for changes in systemic pressure.

Glomerular filtration rate can be measured by inulin clearance. This is because inulin is soluble, freely filterable by the glomerulus and is neither secreted nor reabsorbed by the tubules. Thus the amount of inulin excreted in the urine in a given time will equal the amount filtered by the glomeruli in the same time. The amount excreted divided by the plasma concentration gives the volume of plasma filtrate formed in this time and this is known as the glomerular filtration rate (GFR).

The clearance of a substance is that volume of plasma totally cleared of the given substance in unit time. For inulin the clearance is equal to the glomerular filtration rate but for substances reabsorbed the clearance will be lower than the GFR and for substances secreted by tubular cells the clearance will be greater than the GFR. The inulin clearance of a normal adult is 120 ml/min.

An estimation of the GFR can be made by measurement of the creatinine clearance (*see* Chapter 3). Creatinine is convenient because unlike inulin it is endogenous. It is excreted by glomerular filtration and although small amounts may be secreted by the tubules it affords a useful estimate of GFR for clinical purposes.


## TUBULAR FUNCTION

The glomeruli produce approximately 180 l of filtrate daily. The function of the tubule is to modify this filtrate so that there is an efficient excretion of waste products and a retention of those substances required for normal metabolism. The tubules are able to reabsorb material from the filtrate and to add substances by a process of secretion.

The volume of filtrate is greatly reduced as it passes along the tubule. Approximately 80 per cent is iso-osmotically reabsorbed by the proximal tubule so that only 35 l daily enter the loop of Henle. During passage through the loop further diminution in volume occurs due to the diffusion of water into the hypertonic medullary interstitium. In this way some 15–20 l daily are delivered to the distal tubule. The final adjustments take place in the distal tubule and particularly the collecting duct where water is reabsorbed in the presence of antidiuretic hormone (ADH) to produce a concentrated urine of approximately 1·5 l. Thus the kidney normally reabsorbs in the region of 178·5 l daily.

**Tubular Reabsorption.** The glomerular filtrate contains large quantities of material which are essential for the body and these must be reabsorbed to prevent depletion. In many instances the amount filtered daily far exceeds the total body stores, e.g. sodium. Reabsorption can be active or passive.

Active reabsorption has either a transport maxima (Tm) or a gradient-time limitation to capacity. Substances with a transport maxima (glucose, phosphate, sulphate, lactate, certain amino acids, etc.) are reabsorbed up to a fixed amount of solute in a given time. If the tubule is presented with more than this amount the excess will be excreted in the urine. The renal threshold is that concentration of solute above which the solute spills over and appears in the urine (*Fig.* 2.1). Gradient-time limited reabsorption is dependent upon the gradient which can be established across the tubular wall within the time interval that the filtrate is in contact with the tubular cells. The reabsorption of sodium is limited in this way.

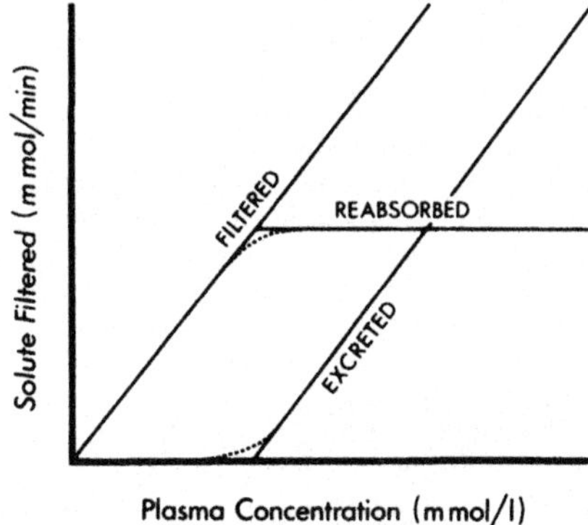


*Fig.* 2.1. Relationship between plasma concentration and urinary excretion for a substance with a tubular reabsorption which has a transport maxima (Tm).

Passive reabsorption occurs by the diffusion of solutes down concentration or electrical gradients. For example water diffuses passively out of the proximal tubule down the osmotic gradient created by the active transport of sodium. Similarly, chloride flows down the potential gradient created by the same mechanism.

**Tubular Secretions.** The tubule can secrete certain substances from the extracellular fluid to the tubular fluid. Three types of secretory mechanism exist:

1. TIME-LIMITED SECRETION. Two appear to be important, one secretes organic acids and certain drugs (thiazides, penicillins), while the second secretes organic bases such as histamine, guanidine etc. The substances secreted by each of these two mechanisms compete with each other for a common transport system.

    2.  GRADIENT-TIME LIMITED MECHANISM. Hydrogen ions are pro-
bably secreted by this means.

    3.  PASSIVE SECRETION. This involves the mechanism of diffusion
trapping, e.g. ammonia diffuses into the tubular lumen and becomes
'trapped' as it forms ammonium which is much less diffusible.

## URINE CONCENTRATION AND DILUTION

In comparative physiology the ability to form a concentrated urine is
associated with the presence of loops of Henle and in general terms the
longer the loops the greater the ability to concentrate the urine. The loop
of Henle thus seems to be important in the concentration of urine and its
special anatomical configuration has given rise to the *countercurrent
multiplier* hypothesis.

In the loop of Henle there is an active pumping of chloride out of the
ascending limb into the medullary interstitium. This is accompanied by the
passive diffusion of sodium ions. The descending limb is relatively permeable to sodium and chloride and thus as the filtrate passes down the limb
its concentration of sodium and chloride increases so that the maximal
concentration occurs at the tip of the loop. As the filtrate passes up the
ascending limb chloride is actively pumped out followed passively by
sodium so that by the time filtrate enters the distal tubule it is relatively
hypotonic. This hypotonicity only occurs because the ascending limb is
impermeable to water. This system provides the medullary interstitium
with increasing osmolality from the corticomedullary junction to the tip of
the papilla. This system is a countercurrent multiplier (*Fig.* 2.2).

Concentration of the urine occurs by the reabsorption of water as the
filtrate passes through the distal tubule and the collecting duct. Under the
influence of ADH the cells become more permeable to water and thus as
the collecting duct passes through the medulla to the tip of the papilla the
osmolality of the filtrate equilibrates with that of the surrounding interstitium. In this way the kidney under the influence of ADH can form
urine as concentrated as the extracellular fluid in the interstitium of the
medulla. In a healthy individual the osmolarity of the urine can be increased
to a maximum of approximately 1200 mosm/l. Inability to form a concentrated urine is therefore found in those conditions where there is destruction
of the medulla, e.g. severe pyelonephritis, medullary cystic disease, nephrocalcinosis. As the maintenance of the hypertonic medulla is dependent on
the continual pumping of chloride out of the ascending limb any process
which stops the flow of filtrate will cause dissipation of the gradient and
therefore results in an inability to form concentrated urine, e.g. in obstructive uropathy, acute tubular necrosis. In these conditions, following
the restoration of renal function there is a diuretic phase which lasts until
the medullary hypertonicity is re-established.

A dilute urine is formed by the hypotonic fluid which enters the distal tubule passing through this tubule without any reabsorption of water. Further dilution may occur if solute is reabsorbed in the distal tubule. In a normal person the osmolarity of the urine can fall to about 50 mosm/l.

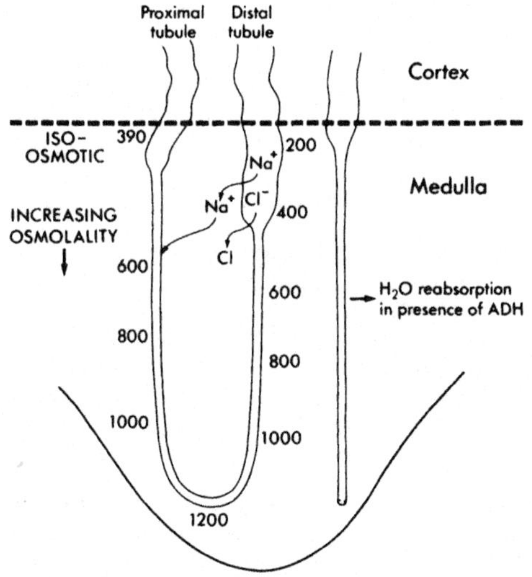


*Fig.* 2.2. Countercurrent multiplier system of urinary concentration. Chloride is actively pumped out of the ascending limb into the interstitium, sodium follows passively. Sodium chloride diffuses into the descending limb and so the osmolality increases to a maximum at the tip of the loop. Urine in the collecting duct is concentrated by the reabsorption of water in the presence of ADH.

## SODIUM EXCRETION

The glomerular filtrate presents the renal tubules with approximately 25 000 mmol of sodium daily which represents an amount in the region of six times the total body store. The average daily urinary excretion is in the range of 100–150 mmol and thus over 99 per cent of the filtered load must be reabsorbed by the tubules. The daily urinary excretion is close to the daily intake.

Sodium reabsorption occurs at various sites in the nephron. In the proximal tubule 65 per cent of the filtered load is reabsorbed isotonically.

In the loop of Henle chloride is actively pumped out of the ascending limb and sodium follows passively (*see* p. 14). Twenty-five per cent of sodium reabsorption occurs in the loop of Henle. In the distal tubule some 8–9 per cent of reabsorption takes place and in the late part of this section it is under the influence of aldosterone. The collecting duct is responsible for the final 1–2 per cent. Sodium excretion can occur over a wide range, less than 5 mmol daily in severe depletion to over 400 mmol daily in excessive intake.

The control of sodium excretion has been the subject of intense study but there are still many unanswered questions. The factors involved are:

1. *Glomerular filtration rate*, as the glomerular filtration rate increases there is not a concomitant increase in sodium excretion. This has been described as *glomerular tubular balance* of reabsorption such that an increased or decreased filtered load of sodium is accompanied by an increased or decreased reabsorption so that the amount excreted remains fairly constant. The mechanism whereby this can be achieved is not known.

2. *Aldosterone*, which controls the rate of reabsorption of sodium in the distal tubule. In hypovolaemia aldosterone secretion is increased due to the action of the renin–angiotensin system. Distal tubular sodium reabsorption is increased and water follows passively and the net effect is an attempt to restore the extracellular volume.

3. *Natriuretic Factor* (*third factor*) is responsible for the increased excretion of sodium which occurs in volume expansion. This substance is probably a polypeptide but its site of production and secretion is unknown.

4. *Plasma Sodium Concentration;* in hypernatraemia there is increased excretion which is not just due to an increased filtered load. The mechanism of this is unknown.

## POTASSIUM EXCRETION

The majority of the potassium filtered by the glomerulus is reabsorbed actively by the proximal tubule. The distal tubule secretes potassium in an amount approximately equal to the dietary intake so that balance is maintained.

The distal tubular $K^+$ secretion is closely linked to $Na^+$ reabsorption and $H^+$ secretion. In conditions of increased sodium reabsorption $K^+$ secretion and excretion are increased. However, when the delivery of sodium to the distal tubule is low $K^+$ excretion is diminished. The distal tubular cell $H^+$ concentration is important in $K^+$ secretion. In potassium depletion there is an extracellular alkalosis but an intracellular acidosis. This results in increased $H^+$ secretion by the distal tubule and an associated decrease in $K^+$ secretion; conversely when total body potassium is high there is a diminution in $H^+$ secretion and an increase in $K^+$ secretion and excretion.

## CHLORIDE EXCRETION

The chloride anion follows sodium during reabsorption. In chloride depletion there is an increase in the amount of sodium reabsorbed in exchange for $H^+$ with the consequent generation of $HCO_3^-$ by the tubular cells. Chloride depletion thus produces an alkalosis but in this way the total anion concentration is kept relatively constant. Conversely the administration of large amounts of chloride diminishes the sodium–hydrogen exchange and there is a consequent alkaline urine and decrease in plasma bicarbonate.

## UREA EXCRETION

Urea is the mode in which the waste products of protein metabolism are excreted. There is no evidence for active secretion or reabsorption of urea in the human nephron. Urea is a freely diffusible substance and its concentration in the interstitium of the medulla increases from the cortico-medullary junction to the tip of the papilla. In this way, under the influence of ADH, the urea concentration of the urine in the collecting duct can equilibrate with the urea in the medulla. Thus there is an efficient concentration of urinary urea without an active urea pump. The maintenance of this method of concentrating urea is, however, entirely dependent on the continued action of the medullary countercurrent system.

## REGULATION OF ACID-BASE

**Introduction.** A normal diet results in the production of approximately 50–80 mmol of hydrogen ion daily and if a stable pH is to be maintained then these ions must be excreted. The role of the kidney in acid-base balance is to:
1. Maintain a normal plasma bicarbonate concentration.
2. Excrete hydrogen ion.
The excretion of hydrogen ion is achieved by three methods:
1. Reabsorption of bicarbonate from glomerular filtrate.
2. Acidification of buffers in the tubular urine.
3. Production of ammonia and excretion of ammonium.

**Bicarbonate Reabsorption.** Approximately 5000 mmol of bicarbonate are filtered by the glomeruli and thus enter the renal tubules daily. Clearly this must be reabsorbed otherwise depletion would occur rapidly. The reabsorption of bicarbonate involves the exchange of sodium for hydrogen across the luminal surface of the tubular cell. The hydrogen is produced in the tubular cell by the production of carbonic acid from carbon dioxide and water and the subsequent action of carbonic anhydrase producing hydrogen and bicarbonate. The bicarbonate and sodium pass through the tubular cell and into the interstitial fluid effectively returning the filtered bicarbonate to the extracellular fluid. The hydrogen in the tubular lumen combines with bicarbonate and again under the influence of carbonic anhydrase produces carbon dioxide and water. The carbon dioxide enters the tubular cell and is thus available for the production of more bicarbonate. This process continues as long as bicarbonate is present in the tubular lumen.

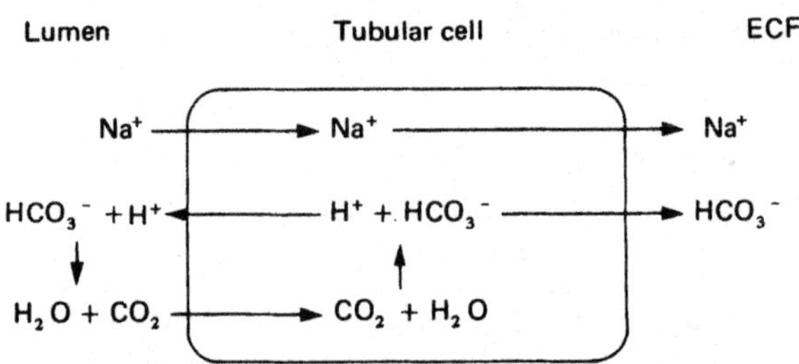


The reabsorption of bicarbonate depends on the plasma bicarbonate concentration. If the plasma bicarbonate is 24 mmol/l or less then effectively all the filtered bicarbonate is reabsorbed and none appears in the urine. When the plasma bicarbonate is greater than 25 mmol/l the amount reabsorbed is constant and the amount excreted increases directly with increasing plasma concentration. In this way the kidney is able to regulate the extracellular bicarbonate concentration. The majority of filtered bicarbonate is reabsorbed in the proximal tubule.

**Acidification of Buffers.** Hydrogen ion secreted by the tubular cells can be buffered by disodium phosphate, hydroxybutyrate and creatinine. The secreted hydrogen is taken up by bases present in the glomerular filtrate and their conjugate acids are formed. The amount of hydrogen ion excreted is limited by the capacity of the buffers but is in the region of 20–40 mmol daily.

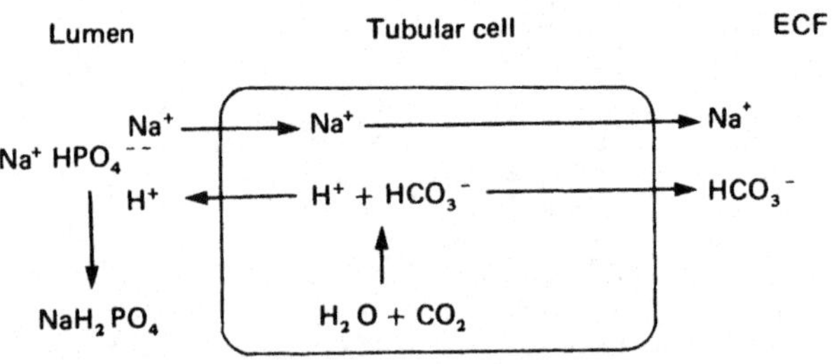

The excretion of hydrogen ions probably occurs throughout the length of the nephron but the buffering by phosphate predominantly occurs in the proximal tubule.

**Excretion of Ammonium.** Ammonia is freely diffusible across cell membranes and that produced in the tubular cells diffuses into the tubular lumen where it conjugates with hydrogen ion to produce the ammonium ion. This ion is relatively non-diffusible and so is 'trapped' in the lumen. Ammonia is secreted throughout the nephron but mostly in the collecting ducts. It is formed in the tubular cell from glutamine although alanine, glycine and glutamic acid may also contribute. The major stimulus to the production of ammonia is acidosis.

**Hydrogen Ion Secretion.** The kidney is responsible for the excretion of hydrogen ion by the secretion of ions from the tubular cells as outlined above. In renal disease this ability is impaired and metabolic acidosis develops. In the neonatal kidney the titratable acid excretion and ammonia production are low and metabolic acidosis may occur more readily. There are several factors which influence this rate of hydrogen ion secretion.

1. *$PCO_2$*. As $PCO_2$ rises the plasma bicarbonate rises due to an increased reabsorption of bicarbonate by the kidney and an increased excretion of titratable acid and ammonia. This is presumably due to the increased production of hydrogen ion in the tubular cell due to the increased $PCO_2$. Conversely as the $PCO_2$ falls there is a reduction in hydrogen ion secretion and a consequent reduction in bicarbonate reabsorption.
2. *Potassium.* In hypokalaemia the intracellular hydrogen ion concentration increases and thus secretion increases. This results in increased bicarbonate reabsorption and a mild extracellular metabolic alkalosis develops. In hyperkalaemia the converse occurs.
3. *Chloride.* Sodium is reabsorbed either with the anion chloride or in exchange for potassium or hydrogen. In chloride depletion a larger amount of sodium will be reabsorbed in exchange for hydrogen and thus there is increased bicarbonate reabsorption with a consequent increase in extracellular concentration, and the development of metabolic alkalosis.
4. *Carbonic Anhydrase Inhibitors.* Drugs such as acetazolamide inhibit the action of carbonic anhydrase and thus reduce the hydrogen ion production in tubular cells. This reduces hydrogen ion secretion and bicarbonate reabsorption.

## AMINO ACID METABOLISM

The kidney is involved in amino acid metabolism by:
1. Conservation of amino acids by reabsorption from the glomerular filtrate. Three pathways exist, the first reabsorbs cystine, ornithine,

arginine and lysine (COAL), the second reabsorbs glutamic acid and aspartic acid while a third reabsorbs the remainder.
2. Transamination to produce certain amino acids such as alanine and serine.
3. Metabolism, by the action of glutaminase on glutamine to produce glutamic acid and ammonia.

## RENIN–ANGIOTENSIN SYSTEM

Renin is an enzyme which is synthesized, stored and secreted mainly by the kidney. Renin-like substances can be extracted from uterus, placenta, brain and adrenals but these probably have no physiological role in the renin–angiotensin system.

Renin is a highly specific proteolytic enzyme which, as yet, has not been fully characterized. It acts on an $\alpha_2$-globulin to produce angiotensin I. This is converted to an octapeptide, angiotensin II, by a converting enzyme which is found in lung, plasma and kidney. Angiotensin II is the main effector substance of the renin–angiotensin system and although it is rapidly destroyed it is a potent vasoconstrictor and stimulus to aldosterone production.

Renin is synthesized and stored in the modified smooth muscle cells of the afferent arteriole which are part of the juxtaglomerular system. The stimuli to renin release are:
1. The tone in the afferent arteriole – a diminution in tone increasing release and vice versa. Thus decrease in renal perfusion due to hypovolaemia and/or hypotension is a potent stimulus to renin release. Impairment of renal perfusion from renovascular disease also stimulates renin release as this simulates hypovolaemia.
2. The sodium content of the distal tubule. It is not known whether the concentration or rate of delivery of sodium to the tubule in the region of the macula densa is the stimulus but it is possible that both are of importance.
3. Mediation by the sympathetic nerves. Stimulation of the nerves stimulates renin release while $\beta$-blockers inhibit this response.
4. Potassium appears to have a slight direct effect with potassium deprivation stimulating release while excessive administration inhibits release.

The secretion of renin is under the control of certain feedback loops:
1. Renin release results in angiotension II production and this stimulates the secretion of aldosterone from the adrenal. This increases sodium reabsorption from the distal tubule resulting in an expansion of the extracellular fluid and a consequent increase in renal perfusion with the subsequent diminution of renin release.
2. The angiotensin II produced has powerful vasconstricting effects and the rise in blood pressure will cause an increase in renal perfusion.

3. Angiotensin II has a direct effect on the juxtaglomerular apparatus.
4. Increase in renal perfusion will increase the glomerular filtration rate and therefore the delivery of sodium to the macula densa, thereby diminishing renin secretion.

The effect of the renin–angiotensin system is therefore a feedback mechanism to maintain blood pressure and renal perfusion.


## ERYTHROPOIETIN

This is a hormone produced by the kidney and which has a regulating role in the production of red cells but not white cells or platelets. It is mainly produced by the kidney although other sites exist as small concentrations can be detected in anephric patients. Its site of production within the kidney is not known but the stimulus to production is hypoxia. It may be extracted from plasma or urine and it has a molecular weight of 46 000. In spite of considerable research no satisfactory method has been devised for extracting or synthesizing this hormone in sufficient quantities to provide for its use in treating the anaemia of chronic renal failure.


## ANTIDIURETIC HORMONE (ADH)

This hormone is a polypeptide containing 9 amino acids. It is synthesized in the anterior hypothalamus by neurosecretory cells and passes along the axons to be released in the neurohypophysis. Antidiuretic hormone (arginine-vasopressin) is very similar in structure and amino acid sequence to oxytocin. Synthetic analogues of vasopressin are available.

The action of the hormone is to increase the permeability to water of the epithelial cells of the collecting ducts. In this way water will pass from the lumen of the collecting duct to the hypertonic medullary interstitium. Thus to be effective there must be a medullary gradient (*see* p. 14).

The control of secretion is by:
1. PLASMA OSMOLALITY. An increase in plasma osmolality is accompanied by an increase in ADH secretion. This will produce water retention by the kidney and so effect a reduction in plasma osmolality with a restoration to normal.
2. PLASMA VOLUME. A reduction in plasma volume either with or without a reduction in blood pressure causes an increase in secretion.
3. BLOOD PRESSURE. Baroreceptors are situated in the carotid sinus and aortic arch. A decrease in pressure is associated with an increase in secretion and vice versa.
4. POSTURE. Changing from the supine to the upright posture is associated with an increased secretion.

## DISORDERS OF MICTURITION

The disorders of micturition can be considered to be of three different
types:

1. Interruption of the afferent nerves as in tabes dorsalis, results in
   abolition of reflex contraction. The bladder becomes distended and
   thin walled. The only contractions which occur are due to the response of the smooth muscle to stretch and are totally inadequate to
   empty the bladder and large residual volumes result.
2. Interruption of the afferent and efferent nerves as in a tumour of
   the cauda equina. The bladder is initially flaccid and distended but
   then some activity tends to return and the bladder wall becomes
   hypertrophied with a resulting shrinkage of the bladder volume.
3. Interruption of the facilitatory and inhibitory pathways from higher
   centres as in spinal transection. The bladder becomes flaccid and
   unresponsive, it is overfilled and overflow incontinence develops. In
   such patients a voiding reflex may be developed and some para-
   plegic patients learn that voiding may be initiated by stroking or
   pinching the inner aspect of the thighs.

# Chapter 3

# INVESTIGATION OF RENAL FUNCTION

Introduction – Urinalysis – Urine microscopy – Blood urea and serum creatinine – Serum electrolytes – Glomerular filtration rate – Renal blood flow and renal plasma flow – Proteinuria – Urinary acidification test (Wrong and Davis) – Urinary concentration test – Split function studies – Renal biopsy – Investigation of renal structure.

## INTRODUCTION

The investigation of renal function and the determination of the extent of functional impairment is important in the assessment of the patient with renal disease. It is important to conduct carefully urinalysis and then to assess systemetically renal function by a series of planned investigations. Frequently it is necessary to repeat investigations at intervals so that the progression of a disease or its response to therapy can be followed.

## URINALYSIS

This has been greatly simplified by the development of suitable 'stix' tests which employ papers impregnated with appropriate reagents and indicator dyes supported on a plastic strip. The commonly used 'stix' tests give protein, blood, pH and glucose.

## URINE MICROSCOPY

Careful microscopy of the urine is a vital part of the investigation of a patient with renal disease. Microscopy is best performed on a fresh mid-stream sample. Normally some tubular epithelial cells and squamous epithelial cells can be seen. Abnormal findings are:
1. Red cells. These may arise from any site in the renal tract but if detected as rbc casts then a glomerular lesion is present. This simple test may prevent unnecessary investigations such as cystoscopy or retrograde pyelography.
2. White cells, either as single cell or white cell casts. These are markers of inflammation in the renal tract but not necessarily bacterial inflammation. Sterile pyuria raises the possibility of tuberculosis or anaerobic infection but may also be found in radiation nephritis and drug-induced nephropathy.
3. Epithelial cells. Tubular epithelial cells are commonly seen and are of no clinical importance. Similarly, squamous epithelial cells may be detected, more commonly in females, and are of no importance.

4. Casts. These arise from the distal tubule and the collecting ducts. Cellular casts are formed from the aggregation of cells in a matrix of the high molecular weight Tamm–Horsfall mucoprotein. Hyaline casts are of little significance.
5. Bacteria, in an unstained centrifuged sample, are best seen by phase-contrast microscopy. The finding of greater than 20 organisms in a high-power field indicates significant infection. A Gram-stained un-centrifuged preparation is also of value and the presence of a single organism per high-power field is significant. Significant infections are usually accompanied by pyuria but this is not absolute.
6. Crystals. Many crystals such as urates are amorphous but some have characteristic appearances such as calcium oxalate (octahedral) and cystine (hexagonal).

## BLOOD UREA AND SERUM CREATININE

The blood urea may be used as an indication of renal excretory function. However, the blood urea concentration depends on a balance between the rate of production and the rate of excretion. The rate of production can be greatly increased in tissue damage, high protein intake and sepsis and thus the plasma concentration will rise although renal function may be un-changed. The plasma concentration of creatinine is much less affected by such changes and therefore is a better indicator of renal excretory function. Creatinine is formed mainly from the metabolism of muscle and the daily production rate is relatively constant in any individual.

The relationship between plasma creatinine and glomerular filtration rate is not linear (*Fig.* 3.1).

## SERUM ELECTROLYTES

The serum electrolytes are not affected to any major extent by renal function until there is severe impairment. The plasma sodium depends to a major extent on hydration although it may be low (115–130 mmol/l) in such states as salt-losing nephropathy, medullary cystic disease and terminal renal failure. The plasma potassium may be low in renal tubular disease and is frequently elevated in renal failure although normal values are found until remarkably late in declining function. The plasma bicarbonate con-centration depends to a major extent on the function of the tubular cells. In many forms of renal disease the bicarbonate falls and this is a universal finding in chronic renal failure.

## GLOMERULAR FILTRATION RATE

There are a number of tests available for the measurement of glomerular filtration rate but the creatinine clearance is the only one convenient for routine use.

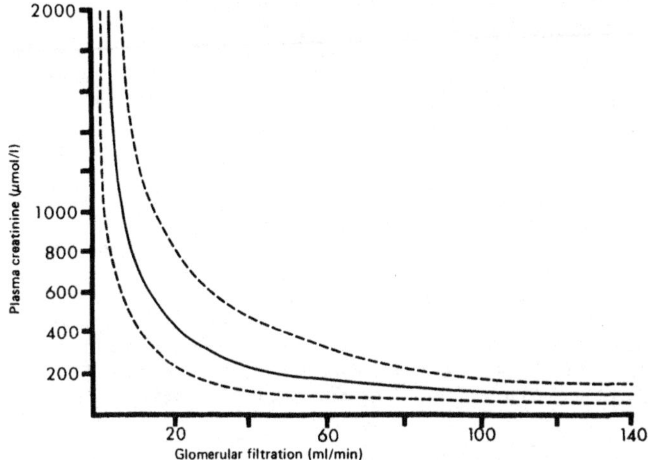


*Fig.* 3.1. Relationship between serum creatinine and glomerular filtration rate.

The clearance of a substance is the volume of plasma completely cleared of that substance in unit time. This is normally expressed as millilitres of blood cleared per minute.

Creatinine clearance gives a good approximation of glomerular filtration rate as creatinine is almost exclusively excreted by glomerular filtration and only insignificantly reabsorbed or excreted by the tubular cells. Creatinine has the advantage of having a fairly uniform production rate in any individual and its plasma concentration is not significantly affected by dietary protein intake. The creatinine clearance can be calculated by the following formula:

$$C = \frac{UV}{P}$$

where C = the clearance of creatinine
U = urine concentration of creatinine
P = plasma concentration of creatinine
V = volume of urine excreted per minute

**Test**
1. Collect 24-hr urine sample.
2. Collect blood sample, usually obtained at the end of the collection.

3. Estimate concentration of creatinine in urine and plasma.

4. Calculate clearance from above formula.

*Normal value:* 120 ml/min (normal adult male). In females the clearance is slightly lower, presumably due to their lower muscle mass, since it is in this tissue that most creatinine is formed. The clearance is frequently adjusted to a 'normal' surface area of $1 \cdot 73 \, m^2$ but this is unnecessary for the majority of patients.

The disadvantages of this test are:

1. The need for accurate timed urine collections. This makes values obtained on an outpatient basis particularly suspect.

2. In the presence of heavy proteinuria the clearance may be falsely elevated.

There is a close relationship between the plasma creatinine and the creatinine clearance and thus for everyday purposes the plasma creatinine gives a good indication of glomerular filtration. This avoids the need for accurate timed urine collections and the error introduced from measuring both plasma and urine creatinine is reduced to that of the plasma estimation alone.

The glomerular filtration rate can also be measured by:

1. *Single shot $^{51}Cr$-labelled EDTA.* This utilizes the fact that the excretion of EDTA is directly related to the glomerular filtration rate and thus the rate of decline of plasma $^{51}Cr$ activity can be used to calculate the GFR. A single i.v. injection of $^{51}Cr$ EDTA is given and serial plasma samples obtained to calculate rate of fall in plasma activity. No urine samples are necessary and so this is a particularly useful technique for children and outpatients.

2. *Inulin clearance.* This requires an infusion of inulin to maintain a constant plasma concentration. It is only of use as a research tool.

3. *$^{57}Co$-labelled vitamin $B_{12}$.*


## RENAL BLOOD FLOW AND RENAL PLASMA FLOW

The renal plasma flow can be calculated from the renal clearance of *p*-aminohippurate (PAH) as the clearance is high and independent of plasma concentration over a wide range of values. If it is assumed that all the PAH is removed from blood in passing through the kidney, then the renal clearance of PAH will be equal to the renal plasma flow. From the haematocrit it is possible therefore to calculate the renal blood flow.

The most accurate method of detecting true renal plasma flow is by measuring the concentration of PAH in the renal arterial and venous blood but this requires vascular catheterization and this is impracticable for routine use. The effective renal plasma flow is measured by PAH clearance and this gives a value about 92 per cent of true blood flow. The difference is due to the fact that about 8 per cent of the renal blood flow passes through non-excretory tissue such as the capsule and pelvis.

*Normal values:*
Renal blood flow 1200 ml/min
Renal plasma flow 650 ml/min

## PROTEINURIA

There is normally a small amount of protein present in urine, up to 300 mg daily is accepted. Amounts in excess of this are pathological.

Routine testing is with Albustix or a 'stix' test employing multiple reagents. These tests are semiquantitative and are extremely sensitive. It is advisable to test the urine on frequent occasions as this may give valuable information on the natural history and progression of the underlying condition.

**Selectivity** of proteinuria is a term used to describe the size of the protein molecules being excreted. In selective proteinuria there is excretion of low molecular weight proteins while in unselective proteinuria there are proteins of all sizes, reflecting the range of proteins present in plasma. It is best remembered by considering that in selective proteinuria the kidney has 'selected' only to excrete small proteins while in unselective the kidney has been 'unselective' in the proteins it passes. The selectivity can be assessed by determining the concentration of a low molecular weight protein (e.g. transferrin) in urine and plasma and comparing it with the ratio of a high molecular weight protein (e.g. IgG) in urine and plasma. A more accurate method is to estimate a range of proteins of varying size but this gives little additional information. Selectivity can also be judged from urinary protein electrophoresis.

**Bence Jones proteinuria** is found in patients with myeloma and is due to the presence in urine of the myeloma proteins. It can be detected by heating urine and observing a precipitate at approximately 40–50°C which redissolves at 80–90°C. On cooling the reverse occurs. Bence Jones proteinuria can be more accurately defined on urinary protein electrophoresis. A monoclonal band can be further characterized by immunoelectrophoresis using specific antisera to heavy and light chains. It is important to be aware of the presence of this type of proteinuria as dehydration, such as in preparation for surgery or intravenous pyelography, is dangerous and may be associated with acute renal failure, usually irreversible, from deposition of the protein within tubular lumina.

**Tamm–Horsfall protein** is a higher molecular weight mucoprotein secreted by tubular cells. It is the protein which binds together the cells which are seen in red cell casts and white cell casts.

**Orthostatic proteinuria** is the presence of proteinuria related to posture. In such patients there is a small but significant increase in urinary protein excretion when upright. It is insignificant but there have been minor glomerular abnormalities described on renal biopsy. The significance of these is not known and long-term follow-up studies are required. It is confirmed by failing to detect protein in a sample of urine obtained after overnight supine rest and the detection of protein in two consecutive samples obtained after getting up and about. A similar, but less common, condition exists where proteinuria is detected after strenuous exercise, while it is absent during normal activities.

## URINARY ACIDIFICATION TEST (WRONG AND DAVIS)

The ability of the kidney to excrete hydrogen ion can be tested by the administration of an acid load. Usually ammonium chloride is used. The ammonium ion is metabolized to urea giving rise to one hydrogen ion for each molecule of ammonium chloride:

$$NH_4Cl \rightarrow NH_4^+ + Cl^-$$
$$2NH_4^+ + CO_2 \rightarrow CO(NH_2)_2 + H_2O + 2H^+.$$

The hydrogen ions so produced are excreted by the kidney.

*Test*
1. Ammonium chloride, in capsular form, in an amount of 0·1 g/kg body weight is ingested over 30–40 min. It is advisable to give plenty of fluid and an anti-emetic is frequently required.
2. Hourly urine samples are collected over the next 6 hours. The urine should be voided into containers which contain enough mineral oil to cover the surface of the urine and prevent $CO_2$ loss.
3. In a satisfactory test the plasma bicarbonate should fall by 2–3 mmol/l indicating adequate hydrogen ion production.
4. In normal subjects the urine pH should fall below pH 5·4. Failure of the urine pH to fall below this value indicates renal tubular acidosis.

In clinical practice it is frequently sufficient to test a morning urine sample. If the pH is 5·5 or less then there is no advantage in proceeding to a formal acidification test as outlined above.

## URINARY CONCENTRATION TEST

The ability to form a concentrated urine depends upon an intact medulla in which a concentration gradient is maintained by the loops of Henle (*see* Chapter 2) and the presence of ADH. This system can be tested by a water deprivation test with or without the addition of vasopressin.
*Test*
1. The patient is given a normal lunch but thereafter no fluid is allowed although a 'dry' meal may be given in the evening.
2. The following morning (i.e. 18 h later) two samples of urine are obtained and the osmolality estimated.

3.  It is also useful to obtain a plasma sample for osmolality at this time.
4.  The test can be repeated but with the addition of vasopressin to distinguish between nephrogenic diabetes insipidus and diabetes insipidus due to lack of ADH.

*Warning*

Care must be taken with this test and a close watch must be kept on the patient. In the presence of diabetes insipidus it may be necessary to terminate the test if the weight loss exceeds 4 per cent of body weight or the plasma sodium concentration rises above 150 mmol/l. Care must also be taken with the administration of vasopressin in elderly patients or those suspected of myocardial insufficiency.

*Normal Values*

1.  After 18 h fluid deprivation the urine osmolality should be 1000± 150 mosm/kg.
2.  In diabetes insipidus values of less than 500 mosm/kg are expected.
3.  In patients with central diabetes insipidus vasopressin should restore the concentrating ability but it may take several days of treatment before a satisfactory improvement occurs as it will take this time to re-establish the medullary gradient.

In practice it is often valuable to obtain the osmolality of the first sample of urine passed in the morning. This will usually have an osmolality of 700–900 mosm/kg and if so then there is no need to proceed to a formal water deprivation test.

## SPLIT FUNCTION STUDIES

These are described in Chapter 6, p. 47.

## RENAL BIOPSY

Renal tissue can be obtained by percutaneous or open biopsy. The percutaneous method using either a Vim–Silverman needle or Tru-cut (Travenol Ltd) disposable needle is most widely used.

Localization of the kidney is by:
1.  Surface marking from a standard i.v.p.
2.  Visualization by contrast injection and X-ray screening.
3.  Ultrasound, which has the advantage of avoiding radiation.

In only exceptional circumstances should solitary kidneys be biopsied. It is advisable to have a platelet count in excess of $100 \times 10^3$ and a normal coagulation screen.

The indications for biopsy are:
1.  To determine the nature of the underlying disease process.
2.  To document the natural history of the pathological process.
3.  To examine the effect of therapy.

The complications of biopsy are:

1. *Bleeding*, usually mild and clearing spontaneously. In some instances may be severe enough to produce clot colic and require transfusion. A perirenal haematoma may develop and this occasionally produces hypertension.
2. *Pain*, usually a mild transient discomfort but in some cases severe enough to require analgesia. This should always raise the suspicion of bleeding.
3. *Infection*, which may occur in the kidney or needle tract and is usually due to skin organisms introduced by the needle.
4. *Arteriovenous aneurysm* formation, a rare and late developing complication.

## INVESTIGATION OF RENAL STRUCTURE

**Intravenous Urography.** This is of particular value in determining the size, shape and position of the kidneys. The kidneys are visualized by giving an intravenous injection of radio-opaque contrast, most commonly an organic iodine compound. This is filtered by the glomerulus and acts as an osmotic diuretic in the tubules. The contrast becomes concentrated in the tubules within 5–10 min of injection and this provides a nephrogram. As the contrast passes through the renal tract the renal pelvis, ureters and bladder can be visualized. Tomography can be added to obtain a more satisfactory view particularly in impaired renal function or in obese and poorly prepared patients.

Good visualization is dependent, to some extent, on renal function. If the renal function is known to be impaired then a double dose or infusion of contrast can be given.

The complications of this technique include:

1. Hypersensitivity reactions to the contrast media.
2. Precipitation of acute renal failure in patients with impaired renal function.
3. Precipitation of acute renal failure in patients with multiple myeloma particularly if dehydration has been employed.

Some common radiological findings are:

*Acute Renal Failure:* poor uptake contrast but a persisting dense nephrogram.

*Chronic Glomerulonephritis:* small, smooth, regularly contracted kidneys.

*Chronic Pyelonephritis:* small, irregularly contracted kidneys with clubbing and dilatation of the calyces and irregular narrowing of the cortex.

*Pregnancy:* dilatation of the upper urinary tract, frequently more marked on the right side and occasionally persisting for many months after delivery.

*Polycystic Renal Disease:* large irregular kidneys with multiple filling defects and stretching of the calyces around the cysts.

*Renal Artery Stenosis:* on the affected side the kidney is smaller, the contrast appears later, becomes more dense and persists longer.

**Micturating Cystogram.** The bladder is catheterized and contrast media is instilled so that the bladder may be visualized. Voiding can then be observed on screening and the degree of vesico-ureteric reflux can be assessed. This is the reflux of urine from the bladder into the ureter from incompetence of the vesico-ureteric valve. The severity of reflux may be graded:

Grade   I: contrast flows into the ureter but does not reach the kidney.

Grade  II: contrast flows into the ureter and reaches the kidney but does not cause distension of the calyces.

Grade III: contrast flows into the ureter, reaches the kidney and causes distension of the pelvis and calyces.

The value of accurate grading is that it affords a means of documenting the extent of the reflux and allows comparison with follow-up examinations, particularly if surgical correction has been undertaken.

**Retrograde Pyelography.** This is the visualization of the ureters, pelvis and calyceal system by the introduction of contrast through ureteric catheters. These are inserted under direct vision at cystoscopy and so it also affords the opportunity of looking directly at the interior of the bladder. It is of particular value in obstructive uropathy and also in the clear visualization of the urinary tract in patients with poor renal function.

The major disadvantage is the possibility of introducing infection to the urinary tract. It also requires considerable skill as it is possible to over-distend the system and so give the impression of hydronephrosis.

**Arteriography.** This is used to examine the arterial supply to the kidney and is of particular value in the investigation of renal artery stenosis. It requires femoral puncture and the introduction of an arterial catheter to the level of the renal arteries. Selective renal artery catheterization may also be performed.

It can be used to define the vascular supply to a space occupying lesion to differentiate between a simple cyst and a malignant neoplasm.

**Venography.** This is used to identify the patency of the renal veins in patients with suspected renal vein thrombosis. It can be performed by a midstream inferior vena cava injection accompanied by a Valsalva manoeuvre or by selective venous catheterization.

**Renography.** This is undertaken by the intravenous injection of $^{125}$I-hippuran and the subsequent measurement of the radioactivity over both kidneys. This provides: (1) a measure of the renal function, (2) a comparison of one kidney with the other, and (3) useful information especially in obstructive uropathy.

The hippuran is rapidly cleared by the kidney by filtration and secretion. A normal renogram shows:

1. A vascular phase as the radioactivity enters the kidney.
2. A secretory phase as the radioactivity becomes concentrated.
3. An excretory phase as the radioactivity diminishes due to urine flow.

In significant vascular disease the first phase is slower in the affected side when compared to normal. In obstruction the third phase is prolonged and the decrease in radioactivity is slower.

**Renal Scanning.** In this technique a radio-isotope is injected intravenously and both kidneys are scanned simultaneously with a gamma camera. The most commonly used isotopes are $^{197}$Hg or $^{203}$Hg-chlormerodrin or $^{99}$Tm-ascorbic acid complex.

It provides good delineation of renal size, shape and position. If computerized facilities are available useful information concerning renal function can be obtained.

**Ultrasound.** This is a non-invasive technique which is particularly useful for determining the size and position of the kidneys. It is capable of demonstrating hydronephrosis and is of considerable value in screening the families of patients known to have polycystic renal disease. It requires skilled interpretation but is safe, non-invasive and can be used repeatedly without risk to the patient.

# Chapter 4

# ACUTE GLOMERULONEPHRITIS

Introduction – Acute glomerulonephritis – Recurrent haematuria

## INTRODUCTION

The terminology in glomerular disease is confusing as it combines clinical and pathological findings indiscriminately. Certain clinical syndromes are recognizable but there is no good correlation between the underlying glomerular pathology and the clinical findings. This chapter deals with the clinical syndromes of acute nephritis and recurrent haematuria. Nephrotic syndrome (Chapter 5) and glomerular diseases, both primary (Chapter 9) and secondary (Chapter 10) will be dealt with separately. It must be remembered that the clinical syndrome does not provide a diagnosis of the underlying pathology although certain associations are well recognized.

## ACUTE GLOMERULONEPHRITIS

**Definition.** A clinical syndrome characterized by the acute onset of haematuria, proteinuria, hypertension and oliguria usually following an infective illness by some 10–20 days. Not all these findings are present simultaneously in all cases.

**Clinical Features.** The syndrome may occur at any age but is most common in children and young adults. There is frequently a history of a preceding infective illness often involving the upper respiratory tract. This may be streptococcal due to infection with a Group A $\beta$-haemolytic streptococcus type 1, 4, 12 or 49 although the incidence of this seems to be declining. Other causal organisms may be found – viral, staphylococcal or pneumococcal but in many instances none are isolated. The clinical presentation is with:

> HAEMATURIA. The urine appears smokey due to the presence of red cell casts. Occasionally it may appear red coloured if haematuria is heavy.
> PROTEINURIA. The amount is variable but is usually less than that required to produce a nephrotic syndrome. It is usually unselective.
> HYPERTENSION. Variable in severity.
> OLIGURIA. This depends to a large extent on the severity of the glomerular lesion.

Other clinical features include oedema due to salt and water retention in the oliguric phase. Encephalopathy may occur and this is due to hypertension, electrolyte disorders (e.g. hyponatraemia) or the deposition of complexes in the arachnoid of the brain.

**Laboratory Findings.** Haematuria in the form of red cell casts (detection requires the examination of fresh urine), proteinuria variable in amount but usually unselective. In the acute phase there may be transient elevation of blood urea and serum creatinine due to impaired renal function. Plasma protein concentrations usually normal. Complement ($C_3$) concentration transiently depressed in acute stage. The ASO titre may be elevated in cases with a preceding streptococcal infection (*Note*, not all streptococci stimulate production of anti-streptolysin O). It may be possible to isolate the initiating organism. Tests for circulating immune complexes may be positive but in a significant number of cases are negative. This is probably due to the relatively insensitive methods and the transient nature of the complexes.

**Biopsy Findings.** There is a wide range of biopsy findings reflecting the fact that a number of primary and secondary glomerular diseases may present as acute nephritis. The underlying morphological appearances may be:

Diffuse proliferative glomerulonephritis.

Mesangiocapillary glomerulonephritis.

Focal glomerulonephritis.

Crescentic glomerulonephritis.

The typical lesion of small soluble complex mediated glomerulonephritis is the finding of subepithelial deposits, 'humps', by electron microscopy. These are aggregations of immune complexes and are most commonly found in early phase of the illness. Immunofluorescence demonstrates these lesions to be composed of antigen, antibody and complement.

**Aetiology.** Most cases are due to the introduction of an antigen with the subsequent formation of antibody and the development of small soluble complexes.

**Pathogenesis.** The lesion is the consequence of immune-complex deposition and the sequence of events is:

1. Introduction of antigen;
2. Latent period of antibody production;
3. Formation of small complexes due to slight antigen excess;
4. Deposition of complexes in glomerular capillary wall;
5. Activation of the complement cascade;
6. Attraction of polymorphs;
7. Liberation of vasoactive amines and kinins;
8. Increase in vascular permeability;
9. Endothelial swelling and proliferation;
10. Platelet aggregation;
11. Fibrin formation.

The outcome of such a sequence will depend upon two factors: (1) the ability of the kidney to remove the products of inflammation by fibrinolysis and phagocytosis, and (2) the continued deposition of complexes. If antibody production is good the period of small complex formation in slight antigen excess will be short and then followed by production of larger complexes with removal by the reticulo-endothelial system and eventual antigen elimination. In such circumstances there will be resolution of the illness and a return to normality. If, however, the formation of small complexes continues or there is deficiency in removal of the inflammatory products then a progressive condition will result.

**Natural History.** This will depend upon the underlying disease but in those cases due to streptococcal antigen or other 'single-shot' circumstances the majority have a typical illness of:

Haematuria, macroscopic for 1–2 weeks, microscopic for a further 1–2 weeks then resolution;

Proteinuria, variable but generally becoming insignificant after 4 weeks;

Hypertension, resolving in 7–10 days;

Oliguria, usually for 7 days, followed by diuresis with associated resolution of any oedema.

In the majority of cases there will be a complete resolution by 4 weeks.

In conditions where the acute nephritis is the clinical manifestation of a systemic disease then the natural history will depend on the nature of the systemic disease.

**Clinical Associations.** The presentation of acute nephritis may occur in a wide variety of conditions including:

Henoch–Schönlein syndrome

Polyarteritis (nodosa and microscopic form)

Wegener's granulomatosis

Systemic lupus erythematosus

**Experimental Studies.** There are numerous experimental models of glomerulonephritis but unfortunately many have little bearing on human disease. Studies have, however, helped in the understanding of glomerular disease and in particular the relationship of antibody response to the subsequent development of glomerular lesions. The introduction of an antigen may be followed by:

1. No antibody response and in such circumstances no glomerular lesions develop.
2. Good antibody production resulting in only a very short transient phase of circulating complexes which are rapidly eliminated by the reticulo-endothelial system and again no glomerular lesion appears.
3. Poor antibody response in which the phase where soluble complexes are present is prolonged. If the complexes are small they will be deposited in the subepithelial aspect of the glomerular capillary wall. Slightly larger complexes will deposit in a subendothelial or mesangial position. In these circumstances a proliferative lesion will develop.

4. If the antigen is introduced repeatedly in small amounts then there is the repeated formation of complexes and the development of a membranous lesion.

## RECURRENT HAEMATURIA

**Definition.** Repeated episodes of macroscopic haematuria frequently preceded by or associated with an upper respiratory tract infection. Episodes may also occur in association with other febrile illnesses.

**Clinical Features.** It is important to distinguish this clinical syndrome from acute nephritis. In recurrent haematuria there is no latent period between the infective illness and the appearance of the haematuria. Macroscopic haematuria appears within 1–2 days of the infective illness, lasts up to 7 days and microscopic haematuria is frequently persistent between clinical episodes.

It occurs most frequently in children and is rare after the age of 40. Proteinuria is mild and oedema rare. Hypertension and renal impairment are both uncommon except when the underlying cause is mesangiocapillary glomerulonephritis. In a number of instances there appears to be a familial involvement. The prognosis is usually good.

**Biopsy Findings.** A variety of appearances may be found and these, in order of frequency are:
1. Mesangial IgG/IgA disease.
2. Focal glomerulonephritis.
3. Diffuse proliferative glomerulonephritis.
4. Mesangiocapillary glomerulonephritis.

# Chapter 5

# NEPHROTIC SYNDROME

**Introduction.** The nephrotic syndrome is a common mode of presentation in a wide variety of glomerular diseases. In itself it is not a diagnosis but a description of a clinical syndrome just as the terms 'acute nephritis', 'recurrent haematuria' and 'renal failure' describe differing modes of clinical presentation.

**Definition.** The nephrotic syndrome is a clinical state which develops consequent on prolonged proteinuria sufficient to reduce the plasma protein concentration to the extent of producing hypoproteinaemic oedema. In the adult patient this requires a urinary protein loss of 5 g daily with the reduction of the plasma albumin concentration to less than 25 g/l.

**Clinical Features**
1. Oedema is the principal feature, and is usually peripheral, involving the limbs. Facial oedema is more prominent in children than adults. In severe cases ascites may develop. There is no good relationship between the plasma albumin and the degree of oedema but in the adult oedema is uncommon unless the plasma albumin is less than 25–30 g/l. Children tolerate a lower plasma albumin before oedema becomes manifest. Patients frequently complain that their oedematous legs are cold and sometimes numb.
2. Proteinuria; patients may notice that their urine appears frothy.
3. Anorexia and diarrhoea may well be due to severe protein malnutrition.
4. Lethargy and tiredness are commonly present.
5. Muscle wasting is probably due to the catabolism of muscle protein in an attempt to maintain the normal plasma protein concentrations.
6. Infections, particularly cellulitis, septicaemia, peritonitis and urinary tract infections, probably reflect the impaired cellular and humoral immunity due to malnutrition. In addition, certain infections, notably streptococcal, spread rapidly through oedematous tissue.
7. Nail changes. In prolonged severe nephrotic syndrome the nails appear white.
8. Hypertension is variable and is to a large extent dependent on the underlying glomerular pathology.
9. Renal failure, too, is variable and depends on the underlying aetiology.

**Oedema Formation.** The formation of oedema occurs due to the accumulation of sodium and water in the extravascular space as a direct consequence of diminution of the plasma protein concentration.
1. Protein loss stimulates an increased production of proteins by the

liver. However, if the protein loss exceeds the ability of the liver to increase protein production there will be a reduction in the concentration of protein in the plasma.

2. The diminished plasma protein concentration reduces the plasma oncotic pressure and thus there will be an accumulation of fluid in the extravascular space. This fluid will originate from the plasma and so will result in hypovolaemia.

3. The hypovolaemia reduces renal blood flow and glomerular filtration thereby inhibiting the secretion of natriuretic factor and stimulating the secretion of renin. The renin increases aldosterone secretion from the adrenal.

4. The hypovolaemia also stimulates the secretion of ADH.

5. The net effect of (3) and (4) is maximal conservation of sodium and water by the kidney in an attempt to restore the diminished blood volume.

6. The retained salt and water, however, pass out into the extravascular space due to the continued low plasma oncotic pressure and thus leads to further accumulation of oedema.

## Laboratory Findings

1. *Urine.* Proteinuria which may vary from 5 to 20 g daily. The protein selectivity will depend on the underlying pathology. Similarly, haematuria may be present depending on the glomerular lesion. Urine microscopy may show hyaline casts, oval fat bodies and occasionally doubly refractile fat bodies.

2. *Plasma Proteins.* There is reduction in plasma albumin and total protein. This may be associated with an increase in the $\alpha_2$- and $\beta$-globulins. The $\gamma$-globulins may be normal or slightly elevated. Fibrinogen concentration is increased.

3. *Urea and Creatinine.* These are frequently normal unless severe hypovolaemia is producing a prerenal failure. If the underlying disease is membraneous or mesangiocapillary glomerulonephritis there is frequently renal functional impairment and thus the plasma urea and creatinine will be elevated.

4. *Lipids.* Plasma cholesterol is elevated and its concentration appears to vary inversely with that of albumin. Phospholipid and triglyceride concentrations are increased. High-density lipoproteins are reduced, probably due to increased urine losses. The $\beta$ and pre-$\beta$ lipoproteins are increased.

5. *Calcium* is low and even correction for the low plasma albumin frequently reveals a true hypocalcaemia.

6. *ESR* elevated.

7. *Platelets* usually elevated and frequently their adhesiveness is increased.

**Complications of Nephrotic Syndrome.** There are many well recognized complications of the nephrotic syndrome and to these can be added the complications of therapy which may be used in patients who are nephrotic.

1. Subnutrition state, which develops as a result of urinary protein loss and the frequent anorexia and diarrhoea which accompanies many instances of nephrotic syndrome. Clinically this is visible by skin changes, osteoporosis and muscle wasting. In addition, the poor nutrition interferes with both cellular and humoral immunity and so infections are common.
2. Bacterial infections, particularly cellulitis, pericarditis, septicaemia and urinary tract infections.
3. Clotting episodes which involve both the arterial and venous systems are due to the raised plasma fibrinogen, Factors V, VII, VIII and X and the increased platelet count and adhesion. Renal vein thrombosis is particularly common.
4. Ischaemic heart disease is probably due to the lipid abnormalities, increased coagulation factors, increased platelet adhesion and the fact that a number of patients are hypertensive.
5. Hypovolaemia may only be manifest as postural hypotension or may be sufficient to cause circulatory collapse and acute renal failure.
6. Secondary tubular disease, amino aciduria and glycosuria may appear.

The complications above may be compounded by complications arising from therapy used to treat the syndrome, its complications or the underlying glomerular pathology.

1. Diuretics may accentuate the hypovolaemia and also produce hyponatraemia and hypokalaemia.
2. Steroids increase the tendency to infection, thrombosis and osteoporosis. In addition, they may produce hypertension, a Cushingoid appearance and growth failure.
3. Cytotoxics increase liability to infection. In addition, they may produce nausea, gastritis, cystitis, hair loss and marrow depression.
4. Antibiotics should not be used prophylactically in spite of the increased tendency to infection.
5. Clofibrate has been suggested as a treatment of the lipid abnormalities but there is a high incidence of disabling muscular complications.

It must be remembered that many drugs are protein bound and so in hypoproteinaemia all must be used with caution and dosage reduction considered otherwise there will be a high incidence of side effects.

**Causes of Nephrotic Syndrome.** A wide variety of glomerular diseases can produce nephrotic syndrome. Approximately 80 per cent are primary glomerular diseases, 18 per cent renal involvement from systemic disease, and the remainder are due to such conditions as infections, drugs, malignancies and rare congenital diseases. Some conditions such as minimal lesion glomerulonephritis are common in childhood while others such as amyloid, membranous glomerulonephritis and diabetic glomerulosclerosis are much more common in adults.

1. *Glomerulonephritis*
   Diffuse proliferative (5 upwards)*
   Membranous (30–50)*
   Mesangiocapillary (15–30)*
   Focal (15 upwards)*
   Minimal lesion (1–12)*
   Focal glomerulosclerosis (5–15)*
2. *Systemic Diseases*
   Systemic lupus erythematosus (15–30)*
   Henoch–Schönlein syndrome (5–20)*
   Diabetes mellitus (30 upwards)*
   Amyloidosis (30 upwards)*
   Sarcoidosis
   Scleroderma
3. *Infections*
   Syphilis
   Quartan malaria
   Subacute bacterial endocarditis
   Leprosy
4. *Drug-induced*
   Penicillamine
   Gold
   Mercury
   Phenindione
   Trimethadione
   Heroin addiction
5. *Malignancy*
   Carcinoma stomach
   Carcinoma breast
   Choriocarcinoma
   Multiple myeloma
   Hodgkin's disease
6. *Renal Vein Thrombosis* (see p. 53)
7. *Congenital and Familial Conditions*

**Management.** The management of the patient should be aimed at:
   1. Symptomatic relief of oedema.
      *a. Diet.* A high protein intake of 1·5–2·0 g/kg/day with a restricted sodium intake, less than 30 mmol/day if possible.

---

*Indicates most common age at presentation.

    *b. Diuretics.* Initial therapy will require the so-called 'loop' agents such as frusemide, ethacrynic acid or bumetanide. In many instances the addition of a distal acting diuretic such as spironolactone, amiloride or triamterene will be required. Once the oedema clears it is frequently possible to maintain an oedema-free state with a reduced dose or a mild diuretic such as a thiazide.

    *c. Albumin.* Infusions of albumin raise the plasma oncotic pressure and thus draw back the oedema into the vascular space. In combination with diuretics this can produce a massive diuresis. However, much of the infused protein is lost in the urine and thus albumin should be reserved for patients with hypovolaemia when acute renal failure may develop and for patients in whom a satisfactory diuresis cannot be achieved by high dose combined diuretics. Some patients can be kept remarkably well with weekly or fortnightly infusions of 40 g salt-poor albumin.

2. Search for known aetiological agents. Appropriate investigations for systemic diseases, malaria, syphilis, drugs and malignancies.

3. *Renal Biopsy.* It is important to determine the underlying pathology so that specific treatment can be initiated if indicated. Biopsy is not without risk and it may be possible to reach a satisfactory diagnosis without renal histology, e.g. a nephrotic child with no hypertension, no haematuria and a highly selective proteinuria is most likely to have a minimal lesion glomerulonephritis. Similarly it should be possible to make a diagnosis of drug-induced cases, diabetic glomerulosclerosis and infection-induced cases without recourse to biopsy. In some circumstances, such as systemic lupus erythematosus a knowledge of the histology is useful in determining prognosis.

4. Treatment of underlying glomerular disease. For some conditions specific therapy is indicated (*see* Chapters 9 and 10).

5. Follow-up. Many patients with nephrotic syndrome run a relapsing and remitting course and so careful long-term follow-up is necessary. The prognosis is extremely variable but the presence of haematuria, hypertension and/or impaired renal function indicates poor prognosis.

# Chapter 6

# HYPERTENSION

Introduction – Classification of hypertension – Essential hypertension – Malignant hypertension – Pathogenesis of renal hypertension – Renin – Saralasin test – Renal artery stenosis – Management of hypertension – Hypotensive drugs – Renal vein thrombosis – Renal infarction

## INTRODUCTION

Hypertension is common and approximately 5 per cent of the adult population have a diastolic pressure in excess of 110 mmHg. The majority have essential hypertension but a significant number have some underlying cause and can therefore be considered as having secondary hypertension. The approximate distribution of hypertension is:

| | |
|---|---|
| Essential | 85% |
| Secondary | |
|     Renal | 10% |
|     Adrenal | 2% |
|     Miscellaneous | 2% |
| Malignant | 1% |

Thus of the various secondary causes underlying renal disease is the most common. In addition, a number of patients with essential and other secondary forms of hypertension will have their illness complicated by renal damage which frequently will further exacerbate the hypertension.

## CLASSIFICATION OF HYPERTENSION

Hypertension may be classified in the following way:
1. *Essential:* no obvious cause apparent.
2. *Renal*
   a. *Vascular*
      Atheroma
      Fibromuscular hyperplasia
      Dissecting aneurysm
      Arteritis
      Embolic
      Extrinsic pressure
   b. *Parenchymal*
      Glomerulonephritis
      Pyelonephritis
      Polycystic disease
      Irradiation injury
      Systemic diseases

      Hydronephrosis
      Segmental hypoplasia
   c. *Tumours*
      Haemangiopericytoma
      Hypernephroma
      Wilms's tumour
3. *Adrenal*
   a. *Medulla*
      Phaeochromocytoma and related neural tumours
   b. *Cortex*
      Cushing's syndrome
      Conn's syndrome
      Hyperplasia
4. *Coarctation of Aorta*
5. *Pregnancy*
   Eclampsia and pre-eclampsia
   Post-toxaemia syndromes
   Postpartum acute renal failure
6. *Malignant (vide infra)*

## ESSENTIAL HYPERTENSION

The majority of patients with hypertension have no obvious underlying cause and are thus termed 'essential'. There is modest evaluation of the diastolic pressure to 90–120 mmHg and the incidence increases with age.

    Renal involvement is not common in essential hypertension although renal arteriolosclerosis may occur. The major complication is the development of left ventricular hypertrophy which may lead to congestive cardiac failure. There is also an increased incidence of vascular disease, particularly atheroma. The cause of death in essential hypertension is:

| | |
|---|---|
| Left ventricular failure | 30–50% |
| Cerebrovascular disease | 10–20% |
| Renal failure | 10% |
| Unrelated to hypertension | 30% |

The high incidence of cardiovascular disease indicates the importance of identifying and controlling blood pressure in hypertensive patients.

## MALIGNANT HYPERTENSION (Accelerated Hypertension)

The term 'malignant hypertension' is used to describe a clinical syndrome consisting of:

*Retinopathy* – haemorrhages, exudates and papilloedema.
*Severe hypertension* – diastolic $\geqslant$ 130 mmHg.
*Fibrinoid necrosis* – of arteriolar walls.

The clinical presentation is frequently due to cerebral symptoms such as headache, confusion, stupor and eventually coma. Many patients present with visual deterioration. Renal involvement at presentation is common and is manifest as proteinuria and impaired function. It is often difficult to determine whether there is underlying renal disease or whether the renal abnormalities are a direct consequence of the severe hypertension.

Malignant hypertension is a medical emergency and the blood pressure should be controlled to avoid the risk of subarachnoid haemorrhage and to preserve vision. Caution must be exercised in lowering the pressure as sudden profound reduction may precipitate arterial occlusion, particularly of the renal vessels, thus producing severe irreversible renal failure. It is adequate to reduce the diastolic pressure to 110–130 mmHg in the first 24 hours and then gradually increase therapy to reduce to 90–110 mmHg by 3 days. The drugs which are most useful are:

1. Hydralazine, 10–20 mg i.m. hourly p.r.n.
2. Labetalol, 50 mg i.v. repeated at 5 min intervals increasing to 200 mg.
3. Reserpine, 0·5 mg i.m. increasing by increments of 0·5 mg to a maximum of 5 mg or until desired effect obtained.
4. Diazoxide, 300 mg i.v. by rapid infusion (5 min.).
5. Sodium nitroprusside, 0·5–0·8 µg/kg by i.v. infusion.
6. Clonidine, 0·15 mg i.m. half-hourly p.r.n.

It is best to become familiar with several of these drugs as not all cases will be controlled by the use of one preparation.

The prognosis in malignant hypertension is poor not only because of the underlying cause of the hypertension but because of the consequences on blood vessels. Most patients die from either renal or cardiac failure. There is also an increased incidence of cerebral complications and the rarer occurrence of retinal atrophy.


## PATHOGENESIS OF RENAL HYPERTENSION

The kidney may be involved in the production and maintenance of hypertension. The mechanism of this is still controversial but probably consists of:

1. Renin–angiotensin system. The control of renin production is discussed in Chapter 2. In renal ischaemia due to either vascular or glomerular disease there is an increased secretion of renin with the subsequent generation of angiotensin II which has vasoactive effects. This is probably the mode of production of hypertension in unilateral disease, particularly renovascular disease.
2. Sodium and water retention. In parenchymal renal disease, particularly if renal function is impaired, there is frequently salt and water retention. Hypertension is present in some 80 per cent of patients with severe renal failure and a number of these can be controlled

with diet, diuretics and sometimes dialysis. The sodium retention is caused by enhanced proximal tubular reabsorption due to diminished perfusion and enhanced distal tubular reabsorption from the secondary aldosteronism induced by increased renin activity.

3. Other factors. There are probably many other factors responsible for renal-mediated hypertension but at present these are conjectural.

## RENIN

The finding of an elevated plasma renin concentration may indicate an underlying renal cause for hypertension. However, caution must be exercised in the interpretation of renin values as there are many factors which influence renin production such as posture, dietary sodium and drugs.

Plasma renin may be increased by:
*Diuretics:* thiazides, spironolactone, amiloride, frusemide
*Hypotensives:* hydralazine, diazoxide
*Antibiotics:* gentamicin
Plasma renin may be decreased by:
*Liquorice*
*Carbenoxolone*
*Hypotensives:* β-blockers, methyldopa, clonidine, reserpine

The most satisfactory method of obtaining a reliable result is to take the plasma sample while the patient is on a fixed known sodium intake, in a fasting state and after overnight recumbency. Drugs known to influence renin production should be withdrawn as follows:

Hypotensives for at least 2 weeks.
Diuretics for at least 4 weeks.
Oral contraceptives and carbenoxolone for at least 2 months.

Obviously the withdrawal of therapy depends on the clinical situation, the importance of the therapy and the importance of the renin estimation. It must be remembered that if femoral vein puncture and bilateral renal venous sampling are performed there is no point if the patient is taking drugs which invalidate the result of the assay.

## SARALASIN TEST

Angiotensin analogues which are effective competitive antagonists of the action of angiotensin II *in vivo* have been synthesized. The most widely used is 1-sarcosine, 8-alanine-angiotensin II, saralasin. In conditions where it is thought that the renin–angiotensin system is responsible for the production and maintenance of hypertension saralasin can be used to inhibit the effect of the angiotensin II thereby causing a reduction in blood pressure.

Two tests have been described and are best performed after dietary

sodium restriction, frusemide the evening prior to test with the patient in a supine position after overnight rest.
1. Infusion of 10 mg/kg/min for 30 min.
2. Bolus i.v. injection of 10 mg over 2 min.

A positive test is indicated by a reduction in systolic pressure of at least 20 mmHg and a reduction in diastolic pressure of 10 mgHg. The exact place of this test in the investigation of the hypertensive patient is not established and it is not invariably positive in cases of renin-induced hypertension. Clearly it requires detailed evaluation.

## RENAL ARTERY STENOSIS

In renovascular disease approximately 70 per cent of patients have unilateral and 30 per cent bilateral disease.

**Aetiology**
1. Fibromuscular hyperplasia (30 per cent of cases). Most common in young females. In many cases it is unilateral when first detected but may progress to bilateral involvement in a significant number of patients. In the renal artery there is the development of a fibromuscular band in the media which bulges into the lumen causing narrowing. The band extends spirally along the length of the vessel and on occasions reaches as far as the interlobar branches.
2. Atheroma (70 per cent of cases). This is most common in middle-aged males. It is frequently bilateral although one side may be more severely affected than the other.
3. Dissecting aneurysm. Only rarely causes hypertension.

**Clinical Findings.** Patients with renal artery stenosis as a cause for their hypertension are no different from other patients with hypertension. In approximately 50 per cent an abdominal bruit is audible and careful clinical examination with auscultation anteriorly, in the flank and posteriorly at the level of the second lumbar vertebra is required.

Patients with renal artery stenosis usually have fairly severe hypertension and often prove difficult to bring under control.

**Investigative Findings**
1. Mild hypokalaemic alkalosis may be present due to the development of secondary aldosteronism as a result of the increased renin secretion.
2. Intravenous pyelography is of value particularly in cases due to unilateral renal disease. The stenotic side shows a *delayed appearance* of the dye which becomes *denser* and *persists longer* than in the normal kidney. It is important to ask for early films, in particular an immediate or 1 minute film. The stenotic kidney may be smaller than the normal unaffected side. Notching of the renal pelvis and ureter may be seen due to the development of collateral blood supply.

3. Renography shows the delayed appearance and a reduced peak of radioactivity on the stenotic side.
4. Split function studies are now rarely performed but they demonstrate the functional impairment of the stenotic side. Two tests are described:
   a. Howard test; considered positive if the stenotic side demonstrated a reduction in urine volume of at least 40 per cent coupled with a reduction in sodium concentration of at least 15 per cent or a concentration of creatinine at least 50 per cent greater than that from the unaffected side.
   b. Stamey test, considered positive if there was 3 : 1 difference in urine flow rates associated with a 100 per cent or greater increase in the urinary concentration of PAH from the affected side.

   These tests are not now widely used as they require bilateral retrograde catheterization and it is not possible to be sure that all the urine draining from the kidney has been collected. They are also extremely difficult to interpret in the presence of bilateral disease.
5. Renal vein renin assay is a useful test. Samples are obtained from the lower inferior vena cava and both renal veins. The ratio of the concentration of renin from the stenotic side compared with normal should be at least 1.5 : 1 to indicate stenosis producing functional effects. In some cases it is useful to sample from segmental veins as only part of a kidney may be ischaemic.
6. Renal arteriography is useful in demonstrating the nature and extent of the lesion. In fibromuscular hyperplasia there is a typical beaded appearance of the main renal artery and this may rarely extend as far as the interlobar arteries. Frequently lesions are bilateral although one side may be more severely affected. Care must be taken with radiological appearances as stenotic lesions are not necessarily always associated with hypertension and thus should be interpreted in conjunction with other findings.
7. Renal biopsy performed on both kidneys shows that in the stenotic kidney the glomeruli appear 'crowded' and there is evidence of increase in size and cellularity of the juxtaglomerular apparatus. This investigation has no place in the routine investigation of patients.

### Management

1. *Medical.* Many patients will have satisfactory control with the use of diet, diuretics and hypotensive drugs. β-blockers are of particular value.
2. *Surgery.* This should only be employed in patients who cannot be controlled by medical means. In atheroma it is possible to perform vein bypass, thromboendarterectomy, patch angioplasty or to insert a Dacron prosthesis. In fibromuscular hyperplasia the kidney can be

removed, cooled and then bench surgery performed on the fibro-muscular band. The kidney is then implanted in the pelvis.

The results of surgery are:

$$\begin{array}{lcl}
\text{Cure} & - & 50\% \\
\text{Improved} & - & 30\% \\
\text{Unchanged} & - & 20\%
\end{array}$$

A number of patients show improvement but later relapse presumably due to extension of the disease or thrombosis of the vein bypass, angioplasty or prosthesis. In patients with bilateral disease surgical treatment of the most involved side can improve the hypertension and result in easier medical management.

**Experimental Studies.** The experimental work of Goldblatt in 1934 showed that constriction of one renal artery produced hypertension in dogs. Since then a considerable volume of work has been published. Experimentally, unilateral renal artery constriction is associated in the acute phase with increased renin and consequently increased angiotensin II production. This produces vasoconstriction and an increase in blood pressure. If the arterial constriction is sustained there is in time a reduction in plasma renin although the angiotensin II concentration remains slightly elevated. This is accompanied by alterations in sodium and water balance thereby continuing the hypertension. At this stage removal of the constriction or the constricted kidney results in a reversal of the hypertension. If the constriction is continued longer then the experimental animal proceeds to a phase where both the renin and angiotensin II are normal but hypertension is sustained and uninephrectomy has no effect on the blood pressure. It is thought that in this phase the hypertension is mediated by factors from the contralateral unrestricted but possibly damaged kidney. These studies are of interest but do not explain many of the findings in human hypertensive disease.

## MANAGEMENT OF HYPERTENSION

Careful management and follow-up is required for all hypertensive patients.

**1. Clinical Examination.** The finding of an elevated blood pressure should be confirmed by repeating the measurement in a calm and relaxed atmosphere. Detailed clinical examination is required paying particular attention to peripheral pulses, abdominal bruits, heart size and fundoscopy. Enquiry should be made regarding oral contraceptives. Enquiry and examination should be undertaken to determine whether there is an underlying cause, e.g. renal disease, Cushing's syndrome.

**2. Initial Investigations.** These should consist of:

Urinalysis
Serum creatinine and electrolytes
Urine culture

ECG

Chest X-ray

These should also be repeated as required to detect the occurrence of deterioration in cardiac and/or renal function.

**3. Detailed Investigations.** The finding of hypertension, particularly in a young person, should raise the possibility of an underlying cause, particularly renal disease. Detailed investigation of all hypertensive patients is logistically impossible and thus should be reserved for:

a.  Young adults, particularly females.
b.  Young adults with severe hypertension.
c.  Children and adolescents.
d.  Patients whose employment is at risk.
e.  Patients poorly controlled on standard hypotensive regimens.
f.  Patients whose clinical examination and/or laboratory findings are suggestive of underlying renal or adrenal disease.

The investigations which are most useful are:

a.  In suspected renal disease, i.v.p. looking for parenchymal disease and unilateral disease, plasma renin (p. 45), saralasin test (p. 45) and the investigations outlined for renal artery stenosis if indicated.
b.  In suspected phaeochromocytoma, urine for hydroxy-methoxy-mandelic acid (HMMA) and a Rogitine test (5 mg phentolamine i.v. producing a fall in blood pressure of 25–35 mmHg within 5 min).
c.  In suspected Cushing's disease, urine for cortisol excretion and diurnal plasma cortisol concentrations.
d.  In suspected Conn's syndrome or adrenal hyperplasia, urine for potassium excretion (urinary potassium loss greater than 20 mmol/day when plasma potassium 3·0 mmol/l), urine for 24-hour aldosterone excretion, aldosterone secretion rate, adrenal venography or arteriography to localize tumour.

The extent to which these investigations are undertaken will depend on the preliminary examination and findings and are clearly not indicated to every patient.

**Control of Blood Pressure.** Hypertension must be brought under control if complications are to be avoided. (The emergency control of malignant hypertension has already been discussed.)

Therapy consists of:

1. DIETARY ADVICE. Excess weight aggravates hypertension and so overweight patients require weight reduction. Sodium intake in most people is determined by habit rather than need and is usually considerably in excess of requirements. Although the exact relationship between dietary sodium and hypertension is not known it is advisable to reduce excessive intake.

2. DIURETIC THERAPY. Diuretics by increasing sodium excretion reduce total body sodium and lower blood pressure. Thiazides also

Table 6.1. Hypotensive drugs

| Name | Proprietary name | Dose | | Side effects |
|---|---|---|---|---|
| *1. Vasodilators* | | | | |
| Hydralazine | Apresoline | e. | 10−20 mg i.m. p.r.n. | Headache, tachycardia, |
| | | m. | orally 50−200 mg | s.l.e., acute rheumatoid syndrome |
| Prazosin | Hypovase | m. | 2−20 mg daily | Headache, sexual dysfunction, dry mouth, first dose phenomenon |
| Diazoxide | Eudemine | e. | 300 mg i.v. rapid infusion | Care required when other hypotensive drugs are being used |
| | | m. | orally 100−200 mg t.i.d. | Diabetes mellitus, sodium and water retention |
| Sodium nitroprusside | Nipride | | i.v. 0·5−8 $\mu$g/kg/min | Avoid in liver failure and prolonged use in renal failure. Requires administration by i.v. infusion and continuous monitoring |
| Minoxidil | Loniten | m. | 5−50 mg daily | Hirsutism, sodium and water retention |
| | | e. | 5 mg increasing by increments of 5 mg 6 hly | |
| *2. Adrenergic Blockers* | | | | |
| $\alpha$ blockers | | | | |
| Phentolamine | Rogitine | | Used for diagnostic purposes | Tachycardia |
| Phenoxybenzamine | Dibenyline | e. | 1 mg/kg i.v. in 60 min | Tachycardia |
| $\alpha$ and $\beta$ blockers | | | | |
| Labetalol | Trandate | e. | 50 mg i.v. repeated at 5 min intervals to a total of 200 mg | Avoid in asthma, in emergency use must be given to the supine patient |
| | | m. | 100−800 mg t.i.d. | |
| $\beta$ blockers | | | | |
| Propanolol | Inderal | m. | 120−480 mg daily | Contraindicated in cardiac |
| Oxprenolol | Trasicor | m. | 160−640 mg daily | failure and asthma. Raynaud's |
| Atenolol | Tenormin | m. | 100−200 mg daily | phenomenon, bradycardia, cardiac |
| Metoprolol | Betaloc | m. | 100−200 mg daily | failure; use with caution in |
| Sotalol | Sotacor | e. | 20−60 mg i.v. | patients with diabetes |
| | | m. | 160 mg daily | mellitus |
| Nadolol | Corgard | m. | 80−640 mg daily | |

| Name | Proprietary name | Dose | | Side effects |
|---|---|---|---|---|
| *3. Adrenergic Neurone Blockers* | | | | |
| Guanethidine | Ismelin | m. | 20—100 mg daily | Postural hypotension, diarrhoea, |
| Bethanidine | Esbatal | m. | 10—100 mg daily | ejaculatory failure, |
| Debrisoquine | Declinax | m. | 20—400 mg daily | muscle weakness, depression |
| | | | | |
| *4. Ganglion Blockers* | | | | |
| Pentolinium | Ansolysen | e. | 2·5 mg s.c. increasing by 0·5 mg till effect | Postural hypotension, constipation, ileus, dry |
| Mecamylamine | Inversine | m. | 5—25 mg daily | mouth, paralysis of visual |
| Trimetaphan | Arfonad | | used for hypotensive surgery | accommodation, interference with bladder and sex function |
| | | | | |
| *5. Centrally Acting* | | | | |
| Reserpine | Serpasil | e. | 0·5 mg i.m. increasing by 0·5 mg to 5 mg | Depression |
| | | m. | 1 mg daily | |
| Clonidine | Catapres | m. | 0·1—0·6 mg t.d.s. | Initial i.v. injection may cause |
| | | e. | 0·15 mg i.v. repeated up to six times in 24 h | transient rise in blood pressure sudden cessation may produce severe hypertensive crisis |
| Methyldopa | Aldomet | m. | 250—2000 mg daily | Positive Coombs in 20% of those on prolonged 2 g daily, 20% of these have haemolysis, depression, sedation |
| | | | | |
| *6. Angiotensin II Antagonists* | | | | |
| Saralasin | Not yet commercially available | | | |
| Captopril | | | | |
| | | | | |
| *7. Afferent Effect* | | | | |
| Protoveratrim | Puoverim | e. | 0·1 mg i.v. increasing by 0·02 mg till effect | |

e. Emergency use.
m. Maintenance therapy.

have a direct effect on the smooth muscle of vessel walls. It is preferable to use long-acting drugs rather than the more powerful 'loop' diuretics.

3. HYPOTENSIVE DRUGS. There is a wide range of hypotensive drugs (pp. 50–51). It is advisable to become familiar with several drugs from each group of preparations because there is no one drug which is universally successful in every patient. It is common to start treatment with a $\beta$-blocker and adding a thiazide if a satisfactory reduction does not occur. However, a number of patients require, in addition, a vasodilator such as hydralazine or prazosin. If this combination is not satisfactory a centrally acting drug, e.g. clonidine or methyldopa, or an adrenergic neurone blocker, e.g. bethanidine, should be tried. The majority of patients will be satisfactorily controlled with these agents but in some unacceptable side effects occur and so other drugs have to be tried until a satisfactory preparation or combination is found. For this reason it is essential to be aware of the range of available preparations.

4. FOLLOW-UP. This is essential to ensure patient compliance with the regimen and also to monitor the development of cardiac and renal complications. Many patients require adjustments to their drug therapy due to many factors such as weight change, dietary alterations, change in exercise habits and alterations in the severity of the hypertension. Regular follow-up is therefore mandatory. Patients can, of course, be taught to take their own blood pressure and keep their own records, thereby greatly simplifying medical supervision.

## HYPOTENSIVE DRUGS

There is a wide range of hypotensive drugs and although many have a principal site of action they may well produce their hypotensive effect by a combination of actions. *Table* 6.1 gives a list of drugs, their proprietary names, dosages and side effects. In view of the continuing proliferation of drugs it is advisable to have a good working knowledge of only a few drugs, preferably one or at the most two from each group, and to differentiate between those used for emergency and maintenance therapy.

## RENAL VEIN THROMBOSIS

**Clinical Features.** The clinical presentation may be either as a sudden onset of severe flank pain or as a gradual development of a persistent, dull aching, non-radiating flank pain. However, the patient may be entirely asymptomatic; one reported series found that 50 per cent at autopsy had been previously unsuspected and another report found a significant number by renography in patients with the nephrotic syndrome but no clinical evidence of renal vein thrombosis. Symptoms probably depend on the speed with which thrombosis occurs and the ability to develop a collateral circulation. On examination the kidney may be tender to palpation. The diagnosis should be suspected in patients who have back pain followed by proteinuria and also patients with proteinuria who have a sudden increase in the amount of protein excreted.

**Investigative Findings.** On i.v.p. there is enlargement of the affected kidney with stretching of the calyces. There may be scalloping of the pelvis from the development of collateral veins. Aortography is of little value but a persistent filling defect may be seen in the venous phase.

Venography, either of the inferior vena cava or selectively of the renal veins, demonstrates the filling defect due to the thrombus. Testicular renography has been used to demonstrate the left renal vein.

**Associations.** Renal vein thrombosis may occur in:
Nephrotic syndrome
Dehydration, particularly children and neonates
Amyloidosis
Diabetes mellitus
Malignancy, from compression or direct invasion of veins
Hypercoagulable states
Trauma

**Management**
1. If suspected, confirm by renography.
2. Anticoagulation, initially with heparin and then indefinitely with warfarin.
3. Thrombolytic therapy by the infusion of urokinase may be of value.
4. Thrombectomy should be considered but the results are disappointing and rethrombosis may occur.

**Renal Vein Thrombosis and the Nephrotic Syndrome.** Renal vein thrombosis is a consequence rather than a cause of nephrotic syndrome. Experimentally, renal vein ligation does not produce proteinuria unless there is contralateral nephrectomy. It used to be considered that renal vein thrombosis produced a membranous glomerular lesion but bilateral biopsy in unilateral thrombosis shows membranous lesions in both kidneys suggesting that the glomerular lesion is probably unrelated to the thrombosis. In addition renal vein ligation does not produce a membranous lesion in experimental animals. It is now considered that the thrombosis is a consequence of the hypercoagulable state that accompanies nephrotic syndrome.


## RENAL INFARCTION

Infarction of the kidney may be due to:
1. Arterial obstruction
   Embolism

      Thrombosis
      Trauma
      Arteritis
      Sickle-cell disease
  2. Venous obstruction (usually only in children)

**Clinical Features.** The clinical features will, to a large extent, depend upon the size of the infarct. In arteritis such as polyarteritis nodosa or occlusion in sickle-cell disease there may be no clinical evidence of renal disease. In occlusion of the main renal artery by embolism or thrombosis there is sudden onset of abdominal or flank pain followed by macroscopic haematuria, fever and malaise. Transient hypertension may occur.

**Investigative Findings.** The intravenous pyelogram may show loss of function of part or whole of the affected kidney. Renography may be of value in the acute phase of the illness. The findings will depend on the extent of the infarction, and arteriography is of value in assessing the severity of the lesion. In time the kidney will contract and become shrunken and may only be detectable by ultrasound or CAT scanning.

**Management.** In cases with complete main artery occlusion there will be cortical necrosis and no therapy has been shown to be of value. If an embolus is known to be the cause of the lesion then embolectomy is of value as there is frequently enough circulation to maintain a viable kidney although an acute tubular necrosis may develop. In incomplete cases infusion of urokinase directly into the involved artery may result in satisfactory restoration of calibre. In polyarteritis therapy is aimed at the underlying disease while in sickle-cell disease there must be avoidance of factors which will precipitate sickling *in vivo* with subsequent vascular occlusion.

# Chapter 7

# ACUTE RENAL FAILURE

**Introduction.** Acute renal failure is a syndrome complex which includes an initiating event, an established period of severely impaired renal function, a recovery phase and finally a return to normal. It may be precipitated in many clinical and pathological situations and it is seldom that two cases are identical. In most instances it requires detailed nursing and medical management, frequently involving all currently available intensive care facilities. It is frequently complicated by sepsis but providing careful attention is paid to detail some 50 per cent of patients survive and return to normal renal function.

**Definition.** Acute renal failure is defined as a sudden reduction in the function of both kidneys with the subsequent retention of producis normally excreted by the kidneys and therefore an inability to maintain the normal phsiological internal environment. It may occur in people with previously healthy kidneys but it is important to remember that it may also occur in patients with pre-existing renal disease.

**Clinical Features.** The clinical features of acute renal failure will to a large extent depend on the nature of the underlying aetiology. Patients may be severely ill with profound hypotension from either multiple trauma or sepsis while other patients may have a fairly mild illness with little constitutional upset. However, the recognized clinical features are:

1. Diminution in urine volume. This is not invariable as it is possible to have a normal urine volume but still have retention of the products normally excreted by the kidney. The quality of the urine is most important and if this is poor then the excretion of waste products will be impaired. Oliguria is the most common feature and is defined as an output of less than 400 ml of urine daily in an adult patient. Anuria is a lack of any significant urinary output, usually less than 50 ml daily. High output failure occurs where there is a loss of urinary concentrating ability, a urine volume in excess of 1000 ml daily and a rapidly rising blood urea and serum creatinine.

2. Uraemia is not a feature in the first few days of acute renal failure but it is apparent within a relatively short period of time in the untreated case. An important pointer as to whether a particular patient has acute or chronic renal failure can be the state of consciousness at a given blood urea concentration. A patient with acute renal failure is more likely to be drowsy when the blood urea reaches 40 mmol/l whereas a patient with chronic renal failure may have only slightly mental impairment with a blood urea in excess of 80 mmol/l.

3. Pulmonary oedema may occur at any stage in acute renal failure but

may also be the presenting feature. This is particularly the case with patients being treated with intravenous fluids if a careful watch is not kept on fluid balance.

4. Metabolic acidosis occurs over the first few days and is clinically manifest by tachypnoea. This of course may be complicated by the presence of pulmonary oedema.

5. Other clinical features will depend to a large extent on the nature of the precipitating factors which produce the acute renal failure.

**Aetiology.** It is usual to consider acute renal failure in three groups, pre-renal, renal and post-renal. This division is based on whether the main component of the initiating event impairs renal perfusion or impairs the ability of the nephron to function satisfactorily or obstructs the outflow of urine distal to the nephron. This division serves only as a guide and it must be remembered that many of the cases of pre-renal failure, if they remain uncorrected for any length of time, may progress to intrinsic renal failure.

PRE-RENAL ACUTE RENAL FAILURE. The causes of pre-renal acute renal failure are:

1. A low blood volume. This may be due to severe haemorrhage, either into the gastrointestinal tract or following trauma. It may also occur in severe diarrhoea and vomiting, severe burns, the nephrotic syndrome and following prolonged nasogastric aspiration, particularly if this is associated with excessive fluid loss from an ileostomy. It is important to note that the fluid loss may not be clinically apparent, as for instance in an ileus or following trauma where blood has been extravasated into tissue spaces.

2. A low effective blood volume. In states of poor cardiac output there will be a reduction in renal plasma flow with its consequent effect on renal function. Septicaemia is also an important cause of a low effective blood volume.

INTRINSIC RENAL FAILURE. Acute renal failure due to direct damage to the nephron may have many underlying causes:

1. Severe trauma with shock.

2. Septicaemia, most commonly Gram-negative septicaemia, but can occur in any sepsis.

3. Nephrotoxins: there is a wide variety of nephrotoxic agents including metals, solvents, diagnostic agents, drugs, insecticides, weed killers and industrial chemicals (*Table* 7.1).

4. Postoperative, this is particularly so if jaundice is present. It is important to note that it may occur in a postoperative patient without other evidence of shock.

5. Obstetric causes include toxaemia of pregnancy, postpartum haemorrhage, concealed accidental haemorrhage leading to disseminated intravascular coagulation, the use of abortifacients and puerperal sepsis.

*Table* 7.1. Some nephrotoxic substances

---

Antibiotics: cephalosporins, aminoglycosides, tetracycline, amphotericin,
   polymyxin, sulphonamides
Analgesics: phenacetin, salicylates
Therapeutic drugs: quinine, barbiturates
Insecticides
Metals: mercury, bismuth, lead, gold, arsenic, uranium
Solvents: carbon tetrachloride, tetrachlorethylene, methyl cellulose
Glycols: ethylene glycol, propylene glycol
Herbicides: paraquat, sodium chlorate
Miscellaneous substances: potassium chlorate, carbon monoxide,
   phosphorus

---

6. Acute pancreatitis. The exact mechanism relating acute pancreatitis
   to acute renal failure is not known but is probably related to the
   hypotension, hypocalcaemia and frequent septicaemia.
7. Acute haemolytic episodes, incompatible blood transfusions,
   infections in G6PD deficient patients, sodium chlorate poisoning.
8. Acute fulminating infections of the renal parenchyma, such as acute
   pyelonephritis. This is a particular problem in patients with diabetes
   mellitus with analgesic abuse and with established chronic pyelonephritis.
9. Glomerulonephritis, particularly rapidly progressive glomerulonephritis, Goodpasture's syndrome, polyarteritis nodosa, systemic
   lupus erythematosus and Henoch–Schönlein purpura.
10. Vascular disorders. These include emboli to the major renal vessels,
   malignant hypertension, sickle-cell crisis and renal vein thrombosis.
11. Disseminated intravascular coagulation.
12. Radiology using contrast media, particularly if dehydration has been
   involved.
13. Myeloma, particularly if the patient becomes dehydrated as for
   instance in preparation for an i.v.p.
14. Crush injury and non-traumatic rhabdomyolysis.

The above list is by no means exhaustive and serves to illustrate the
many ways in which the nephron may be damaged sufficiently to produce
intrinsic acute renal failure.

POST-RENAL ACUTE RENAL FAILURE. In this condition there is
   obstruction to urine flow and this may occur anywhere from the
   opening of the collecting duct into the pelvis of the kidney to the
   tip of the urethra. It may be produced by obstruction within the
   lumen of the ureter or urethra, it may be due to lesion in the wall of
   the ureter or it may be due to external compression of the drainage
   tract.
1. Renal tract calculi may obstruct the ureter and if this is bilateral will

produce acute renal failure. Calculi, however, may also obstruct at the urethral outflow from the bladder and produce acute renal failure.

2. Lesions within the wall of the ureter, tuberculous glands at the vesico-ureteric orifice may produce compression of the ureter and subsequent obstruction.

3. Extrinsic pressure on the drainage tract may arise from retroperitoneal fibrosis or may also be due to extension of local malignancies within the pelvis.

**Pathogenesis.** In spite of considerable work in experimental models and numerous observations in clinical situations the pathophysiology of oliguric acute renal failure is still uncertain. Tubular and vascular mechanisms have been postulated but it is highly likely that acute tubular necrosis does not result from a single factor but rather the consequence of several, probably inter-related, events.

Tubular mechanisms:

1. Obstruction due to swelling of tubular epithelial cells or from impaction of desquamated necrotic cells.

2. Tubular 'leak' or back diffusion of glomerular filtrate due to destruction of tubular basement membrane.

Vascular mechanisms:

1. Renal ischaemia from reduction in renal blood flow, particularly the cortical blood flow, due to arteriolar vasoconstriction.

2. Suppression of glomerular filtration due to afferent arteriolar vasoconstriction with efferent vasodilatation perhaps mediated by renin.

3. Suppression of glomerular filtration due to alteration in glomerular capillary wall from endothelial cell swelling and fibrin deposition.

4. Shunting of renal blood flow away from the cortex.

**Diagnosis.** The diagnosis of acute renal failure is made by the association of clinical features together with the following findings:

1. Decreasing urine volume, already discussed.

2. Urine sodium, creatinine and osmolality changes. In pre-renal acute renal failure there is a small volume of highly concentrated urine whereas in established intrinsic failure there is a low volume of poorly concentrated urine.

|  | *Pre-renal* | *Established* |
|---|---|---|
| Volume | low | low |
| Osmolality | > 600 | < 400 |
| Sodium | < 20 mmol/l | > 70 mmol/l |
| Creatinine | > X 10 plasma concentration | < X 6 plasma concentration |

These findings can be of considerable help in the management of the new patient.

3. Blood urea and/or creatinine concentration may not be very helpful but the rate of increase, determined by sequential estimation, is of importance.
4. Radiology may be of considerable value in establishing a diagnosis and also in giving some idea of aetiology. Several patterns are recognized: an immediate dense persisting nephrogram is suggestive of acute tubular necrosis, a slowly developing nephrogram becoming increasingly dense with time is suggestive of obstruction or severe ischaemia, and the absence of a nephrogram suggests renal infarction or a severe anuric glomerulonephritis. In addition, changes indicative of chronic renal failure may be detected. In some patients a nephrogram develops very slowly and so it is advisable to obtain a 24-hour film.
5. Pelvic examination is vital in the initial clinical examination as pelvic carcinoma must not be overlooked.
6. Clinical examination and investigation to determine whether there is any evidence of chronic renal failure (pp. 66–72).
7. A careful and detailed history and clinical examination. This may be difficult in the uraemic patient and it may be necessary to obtain corroborative details from relatives.

**Management.** The management of the patient with acute renal failure falls into four distinct parts: the emergency resuscitation, the management of pre-renal or incipient failure, the management of the established intrinsic failure and finally the care required in the recovery phase.
A. Many patients with acute renal failure are severely ill and pulmonary oedema and hyperkalaemia are common. The first aspect of management is therefore to prevent the patient dying from such treatable conditions.
1. Emergency treatment of shock if present. The use of central venous pressure monitoring is frequently necessary to prevent fluid overload. The fluids used will be dictated by the clinical condition, whole blood, plasma or crystalloids.
2. Estimate blood urea and electrolytes. Treat hyperkalaemia by i.v. 50 ml of 50 per cent dextrose and 10 u soluble insulin. Calcium resin either orally or rectally may also be of value. If hyperkalaemia persists then dialysis may be necessary.
3. Chest X-ray and blood gas analysis if indicated. Pulmonary oedema will aggravate the problems of hyperkalaemia and in profound cases may require ventilation.
B. The next phase is to establish the underlying aetiology and determine whether pre-renal, intrinsic, or post-renal failure is present.
1. Full detailed clinical examination and careful history. If cause not obvious enquire about the ingestion (deliberate or otherwise) of nephrotoxic substances.
2. Correct any treatable condition, i.e. infection, cardiac failure.

3. Urinalysis, if there is evidence of pre-renal failure (Na<20 mmol/l, osmolality >600 mosm/kg, urine/plasma ratio for urea X 10) then volume expansion providing no evidence of cardiac failure exists. Mannitol (100 ml 20 per cent) may be infused with or without the addition of a diuretic. Any diuresis which follows requires careful volume replacement. In patients with adequate volume expansion a trial of high-dose frusemide may be of value. Up to 2 g in 24 h may be used but an infusion rate should not exceed 250 mg/h or tinnitus may be troublesome. It is not advisable to use such doses in combination with cephalosporins.

4. If there is any suggestion of an obstructive uropathy then urgent cystoscopy and retrograde catheterization are required. Obstruction may be suggested from the detection of calculi on a plain film of the abdomen. If a complete obstruction is relieved then there may be a considerable diuresis requiring careful fluid and electrolyte replacement.

5. If the aetiology is not obvious this may be because the patient has an acute presentation of the terminal phase of longstanding renal disease. In such patients an X-ray of hands on fine grain film might show evidence of subperiosteal erosions, loss of tufts of terminal phalanges and/or vascular calcification.

6. Urine microscopy should be carried out on all patients as the finding of red cell casts is highly suggestive of a glomerular lesion such as rapidly progressive (crescentic) glomerulonephritis or microscopic polyarteritis.

C. In the established phase management is directed at:

1. Fluid balance. The patient should be allowed a volume equivalent to the urine output plus 600 ml daily. However, note must be taken of all fluid loss from the body by nasogastric aspiration, ileostomy or colostomy, diarrhoea, and/or from the skin by sweating. Additional losses will occur in ileus, severe peritonitis and in patients with prolonged pyrexia. There is thus no simple formula for replacement other than a careful and detailed assessment of fluid loss with the addition of an amount of insensible loss. Daily weighing of the patient is of considerable help.

2. Electrolyte control. The patient must be maintained on a low sodium and low potassium diet.

3. Protein intake. The daily intake of protein should never be less than 20 g. An intake of 40 g daily is to be preferred and if this is not possible due to anorexia or gastrointestinal problems then parenteral nutrition is required. A daily intake of greater than 2000 calories must be achieved. In cases with severe infection or severe trauma an even greater intake will be required.

4. Dialysis. Peritoneal and haemodialysis both have a place in acute renal failure. The indications for peritoneal dialysis are a low cardiac

output, poor peripheral vessels and as a preparation for anaesthesia in a patient requiring surgery for an obstructive uropathy. Haemodialysis is clearly indicated in the case with a rapidly rising blood urea, recent abdominal surgery and severe infections.

The disadvantages of peritoneal dialysis are the potential hazard of puncturing bowel with subsequent peritonitis, puncturing blood vessels, the possibility of developing hypostatic pneumonia from immobilization and 'splinting' the diaphragm, the introduction of infection by the cannula, and the loss of approximately 20 g of protein daily into the dialysate. The advantages are the rapid control of fluid overload and/or hyperkalaemia with minimum discomfort to the patient, the simplicity of the equipment and the effectiveness in correcting the disordered biochemistry.

The disadvantages of haemodialysis are the requirement of good vascular access, the need for expensive and highly technical apparatus, the need for highly trained staff, the rapid fluid shifts which may occur and the need for heparinization. The advantages are the very effective control of the blood chemistry, the allowance of a more liberal diet to the patient, the limitation of active therapy to 4 or 6 hours daily and the better patient acceptability.

The frequency of haemodialysis is determined by the rate of rise of the blood urea, the degree of difficulty in controlling hyperkalaemia and the requirement for fluid removal.

5. Frequent monitoring for infection, daily blood culture is advisable as the signs of infection may be masked by the uraemia.

6. Physiotherapy, particularly to chest to avoid infection and to the limbs to prevent loss of muscle mass.

D. The recovery phase normally occurs after 14–21 days oliguria. However, it may occur even after 6 weeks. During the phase attention must be paid to:

1. Fluid balance. The recovery phase is also known as the 'diuretic phase' due to the fact that the urine output rises from around 400 ml daily to commonly 4 l or more. Hypovolaemia may therefore occur if there is not adequate fluid replacement.

2. Electrolyte balance. Hypokalaemia is common and potassium supplements may be required for a short time.

**Complications.** The patient with acute renal failure is uraemic in spite of either haemodialysis or peritoneal dialysis and thus is liable to develop complications from this. In addition, he is liable to all the complications of the underlying illness as well as those of any patient who is severely ill for any length of time.

1. Infection, particularly pneumonia, abdominal sepsis and septicaemia, may occur. This in part is due to suppression of polymorph function from uraemia.

   2. Gastrointestinal haemorrhage may occur from platelet deficiency, numeral and functional, and also from mucosal damage if profound shock has been present.
   3. Failure to heal wounds.
   4. Deep venous thrombosis which may be complicated by pulmonary embolism.
   5. Pulmonary oedema if strict control of fluid balance is not maintained.

**Prognosis.** The prognosis in acute renal failure is to a large extent dependent upon the cause of the condition and also on the development of complications during oliguria. Untreated cases have a mortality in excess of 90 per cent. Most units now experience a mortality of about 50 per cent. Factors which appear to affect prognosis adversely are:
   1. Age. Generally the older patient has a worse prognosis.
   2. Infection. Whether this precedes or occurs during the illness.
   3. Aetiology. Obstetric cases have a good prognosis, >80 per cent survival; multiple trauma and acute pancreatitis have a poor prognosis <25 per cent survival.
   4. Gastrointestinal bleeding. This may occur due to haemostatic problems or may arise due to mucosal damage from severe shock.
   5. Severe underlying or associated disease.

It is interesting that there has been little change in mortality over the past fifteen years. This is largely due to better management and resuscitation of patients at risk, the widespread use of central venous pressure monitoring with consequent improved control of the circulating blood volume and better antibiotic therapy reducing the number of patients developing acute renal failure but this is offset by the increasing age of many surgical patients, the more strenuous efforts at resuscitation in severely ill patients and the emergence of antibiotic-resistant organisms.

**Renal Biopsy in Acute Renal Failure.** The indications for renal biopsy in acute renal failure are:
   1. Acute renal failure presenting without an obvious cause.
   2. Evidence or suspicion of a systemic disease such as polyarteritis nodosa or other connective tissue disease.
   3. An atypical clinical course.
   4. A suspicion that acute cortical necrosis may be present.
The biopsy findings in patients with acute renal failure are:
   1. Acute tubular necrosis. The appearances will depend upon the stage in the natural history of this condition at which a biopsy is performed. The typical appearances on light microscopy in the established case are relatively normal glomeruli, tubules dilated and lined by flattened epithelial cells, tubular lumina filled with desquamated cells and casts, tubular epithelial cells with mitotic figures, disruption of the tubular basement membrane, oedema of the interstitium, inflammatory cells in the expanded interstitial space

(lymphocytes, mononuclear cells, plasma cells and occasionally polymorphs) and the presence of nucleated cells in the vasa recta of the medulla.

Electron microscopy reveals the same findings except that lesions in the glomeruli, swelling of endothelial cells and fibrin deposition, are seen. Immunofluorescence microscopy is unremarkable apart from generalized staining of the interstitium with fibrin/fibrinogen antiserum.

2. Cortical necrosis. This may be patchy or extend to destroy practically the whole of the cortex. On light microscopy there is necrosis of the glomerular and tubular cells with loss of normal intracellular architecture and nuclear lysis, necrotic blood vessels which may contain thrombosis and interstitial oedema with occasionally some inflammatory cell infiltrate. In long-standing cases of cortical necrosis calcification may occur.

3. Glomerulonephritis. A wide variety of forms of glomerulonephritis may present as acute renal failure:

    Rapidly progressive proliferative glomerulonephritis
    Goodpasture's syndrome
    Acute proliferative glomerulonephritis
    Henoch–Schönlein purpura
    Microscopic polyarteritis
    Systemic lupus erythematosus

4. Vascular disease:

    Malignant hypertension
    Polyarteritis nodosa
    Scleroderma

## DISTINCTION BETWEEN ACUTE RENAL FAILURE AND CHRONIC RENAL FAILURE

Many patients with chronic renal failure have a slowly progressive illness which does not become symptomatic until there are gross metabolic disturbances. It is therefore sometimes difficult to distinguish between acute renal failure and a patient presenting acutely in the terminal phase of chronic renal failure. It is important to make the distinction because the management is different and while all patients with acute renal failure (with few exceptions) require urgent active treatment those with chronic renal failure must satisfy the criteria for suitability for long-term haemodialysis and/or transplantation.

Evidence of pre-existing renal disease is suggested by:

1. A family history of polycystic disease or glomerulonephritis.
2. A history of analgesic abuse.
3. A history of renal disease, e.g. repeated episodes of urinary tract infection in childhood.

4.  The presence of a normochromic normocytic anaemia.
5.  Evidence of hyperparathyroidism, probably best detected by a fine grain film of hands showing erosions, vascular calcification and/or metastatic calcification.
6.  Only mild cerebral depression in spite of grossly elevated blood urea and very low bicarbonate.
7.  Recent therapy with tetracycline.
8.  Failure of development of secondary sex characteristics and stunting of growth.
9.  The finding of bilaterally small kidneys on abdominal X-ray.

## HAEMOLYTIC URAEMIC SYNDROME

This is a syndrome of acute renal failure and microangiopathic haemolytic anaemia. It was originally recognized as a severe oliguric or anuric renal failure but it is now recognized to have a spectrum of severity and mild non-oliguric cases have been reported. It occurs most frequently in children with a peak incidence in patients under 3 years old although it is well recognized in older children and adults.

Frequently the syndrome is associated with a preceding diarrhoeal illness, viral or rickettsial infection. There appears to be a seasonal incidence with most occurring in late spring and early summer. There is often geographical clustering suggestive of a localized infective agent such as a virus. Clinically there is a wide spectrum but purpura and bruising are common features. In severe cases there is multisystem involvement with neurological complications such as coma, convulsions, paresis and retinal changes, and cardiovascular complications such as cardiac failure and pericarditis.

A microangiopathic haemolytic anaemia is present with the blood film showing red cell fragmentation. In severe cases there is a consumption of coagulation factors and a marked diminution in platelets. The renal biopsy demonstrates a variable amount of fibrin deposition in glomerular capillary walls depending on the severity of the lesion.

The management is that of acute renal failure. There is no good evidence that anticoagulation or fibrinolytic drugs have any part in the treatment of the majority of patients although heparin may have a place in severe cases with massive consumption coagulopathy. The prognosis is good with better than a 95 per cent survival with a return to normal renal function.

# Chapter 8

# CHRONIC RENAL FAILURE

**Aetiology.** Chronic renal failure may be caused by any condition which destroys the normal renal architecture. In many patients the underlying disease will be compounded by hypertension which frequently occurs in renal failure. Conditions leading to end-stage renal failure include:

1. Congenital disease; polycystic disease, hypoplasia, nephronopthisis, Alport's syndrome.
2. Glomerulonephritis; proliferative, mesangiocapillary, membranous, focal glomerulosclerosis and secondary conditions such as polyarteritis and lupus erythematosus.
3. Hypertension.
4. Infections; pyelonephritis, tuberculosis.
5. Interstitial disease; analgesic nephropathy, drug sensitivities.
6. Systemic disease, diabetes mellitus, SLE, polyarteritis, scleroderma.
7. Urinary tract obstruction; calculi, retroperitoneal fibrosis.

The above list is by no means exhaustive but serves to provide a framework for considering patients with renal failure. To maintain satisfactory renal function there is a requirement for adequate renal perfusion, glomerular filtration, tubular reabsorption and secretion, and drainage of urine from the kidney by ureter, bladder and urethra. Significant destruction of any one of these processes will lead to renal failure.

**Uraemia.** This is a syndrome which develops as a consequence of a significant reduction in renal function and is due to the resultant impairment of renal excretory, metabolic, endocrine and homeostatic functions. The syndrome complex consists of anaemia, osteodystrophy, neuropathy, acidosis, and is frequently accompanied by hypertension, susceptibility to infection and generalized deterioration in organ function.

**Pathogenesis.** In spite of very considerable research the nature of the uraemic toxin or toxins is not known. Certain substances are known to be toxic and many others are or have been suspected. Almost any substance which is present in abnormal concentrations in patients with uraemia has been suspected as the cause of the syndrome. It is likely that uraemia is caused by the accumulation of a number of substances and it is highly unlikely that any single factor is responsible for the many abnormalities which develop.

The suggested toxins are:

1. Water.
2. Electrolytes: sodium, potassium, hydrogen ion.
3. Phosphate.
4. Parathyroid hormone.
5. Renin.

6. Urea and creatinine (in experimental situations urea is only toxic in very high concentrations).
7. Guanidines.
8. Phenols.
9. Indoles.
10. Middle molecules: these are substances of a molecular weight of 600–1300 daltons and are probably polypeptides.

The search for uraemic toxins is difficult as there is no acceptable method of assaying the biological toxicity of the substances under investigation. However, the identification of the toxin(s) is important as it may lead to the development of better methods of controlling uraemia and perhaps the development of more selective dialysers designed to remove the toxic materials.

**Symptoms.** Many patients remain asymptomatic until they develop severely impaired renal function, i.e. a creatinine clearance of less than 10 ml/min. Seldom are symptoms directly referable to the renal tract and frequently patients will attribute their symptoms to 'getting older' or some other rationalization. The most frequent symptoms are:
1. Loss of energy and weakness due to anaemia.
2. Breathlessness from anaemia and possible hypertensive cardiac disease.
3. Anorexia and nausea due to uraemia and disordered intestinal motility.
4. Headache and visual disturbance due to hypertension.
5. Pruritus from metastatic calcification.
6. Pallor and pigmentation.
7. Loss of libido.
8. A vague feeling of ill health and of 'slowing-up'.

It can be seen that these symptoms are non-specific and generally are produced by the complications of uraemia. They do not point to disease of the renal tract and thus may be misinterpreted. The simultaneous occurrence of more than one of these symptoms should alert the practitioner to the possibility of renal failure.

**Clinical Features**

ANAEMIA. This is a common feature of chronic renal failure. The severity follows the degree of impairment of renal function but in some patients, notably those with polycystic renal disease, it may only appear as a late feature. The cause is multifactorial:
1. Dietary intake of iron and other essential factors may be impaired due to anorexia or the dietary restrictions imposed during conservative management. In the latter case iron and vitamin supplements should be prescribed.
2. The intestinal absorption of iron may be impaired, this is contro-

versial but some degree of malabsorption probably occurs in most patients.

3. Diminished erythropoiesis in the marrow. This has been attributed to lack of erythropoietin but it is more likely due to the toxic effects of uraemia on the marrow precursor cells.
4. Reduced red cell survival.
5. Increased blood loss due to capillary fragility and poor platelet function.

These factors exist in all patients but in any given patient one may predominate.

The management of the anaemia is difficult and as yet there is no real satisfactory treatment. Improvement can, however, be brought about by:

1. Restricting blood sampling to the minimum compatible with good patient care.
2. Iron supplements, either as ferrous sulphate 200 mg t.d.s. or as a once daily slow release preparation.
3. Vitamin supplements, particularly B complex and folic acid.
4. Androgens have been used but their side effects make them unsuitable for routine use.
5. Cobalt is thought to produce mild cellular anoxia with subsequent increased r.b.c. production. It is, however, of no proven value.

RENAL OSTEODYSTROPHY. This is the name given to the bone disease which accompanies chronic renal failure and it is a mixture of osteomalacia, hyperparathyroid bone disease (osteitis fibrosa cystica), osteoporosis and osteosclerosis. In any particular patient one of these processes may predominate but all are likely to be present to some extent.

*Osteomalacia* is the accumulation of osteoid as a result of defective mineralization. This is a consequence of vitamin D deficiency which develops due to reduction in hydroxylation of cholecalciferol. Normally the hydroxylation takes place in the kidney by the action of 1α-hydroxylase but the activity of this enzyme is considerably reduced in renal failure. In this way vitamin D deficiency develops and results in osteomalacia and rickets. In addition it is highly likely that uraemia is accompanied by the accumulation of factors which directly inhibit the action of vitamin D on bone and impair the calcification of osteoid. The nature of these inhibiting factors is not known.

*Hyperparathyroid bone disease* (osteitis fibrosa cystica) is due to the secondary hyperparathyroidism which develops in renal failure. The stimulus to this is the reduction in plasma ionized calcium which occurs due to:

1. Impaired intestinal absorption of calcium as a result of impaired vitamin D activity, and

2.  Increased concentration of complexed calcium as a result of increased plasma phosphate.

The reduction in ionized calcium increases the secretion of parathyroid hormone from the parathyroid glands and this promotes bone reabsorption in an attempt to restore the plasma ionized calcium concentration. In some patients the stimulus to the parathyroid glands may be so sustained that tertiary hyperparathyroidism develops. In such cases the glands, or more commonly single gland, hypertrophy and become autonomous secreting hormone without regard to the plasma calcium concentration. In these patients severe bone fibrosis and cyst formation may occur.

*Osteoporosis* occurs in many patients and may be due to the mild malnutrition which frequently accompanies chronic renal failure and/or due to the endocrine malfunction which is a fairly universal finding.

*Osteosclerosis* occurs mainly in the vertebrae, pelvis, femoral heads and humeral heads. It has also been described in the base of the skull. The pathogenesis is unknown.

The management of osteodystrophy is aimed at controlling the plasma calcium and phosphate concentrations as near normal as possible.

1.  Plasma calcium is best maintained in the normal range. This is achieved by control of the plasma phosphate and by correcting the malabsorption of calcium with vitamin D. The synthetic analogue, one alpha, is at present the most suitable preparation as any induced hypercalcaemia rapidly reverts on stopping the drug, unlike previous preparations with which hypercalcaemia persists for months. The dose of one alpha is in the range of $0.25-1$ $\mu$g daily, can only be determined by trial and must be kept under constant review.

2.  Plasma phosphate is controlled by the use of phosphate-binding agents such as aluminium hydroxide. Care must be taken to avoid hypophosphataemia as this may aggravate the osteomalacia. The aluminium content of these drugs may present a problem with toxicity.

3.  Osteomalacia may respond to vitamin D but there is evidence of vitamin D resistance in such patients possibly due to inhibitory factors in uraemia.

4.  Hyperparathyroidism is managed by attempting to maintain the plasma calcium within the normal range. In this way it is hoped that the stimulus to the parathyroid glands will be normal and so excess secretion avoided. In patients with established hyperparathyroid bone disease a satisfactory response is usually obtained from vitamin D or one alpha. In tertiary hyperparathyroidism it

is sometimes necessary to undertake surgical removal of the autonomous gland. This is indicated when the plasma calcium is persistently elevated, there is evidence of severe hyperparathyroid bone disease and metastatic calcification becomes a serious risk. Plasma parathyroid hormone concentrations are difficult to interpret due to the problems of assay in uraemic plasma. Localization of the hyperplastic gland can sometimes be made by selective venous sampling from veins draining the parathyroid glands.

5. Osteoporosis responds poorly but it is advisable to maintain a satisfactory calcium intake.

6. Osteosclerosis has no satisfactory treatment.

NEUROPATHY. Neuropathy involving the peripheral motor and sensory nerves as well as the autonomic nerves is common in uraemia. The pathogenesis of the impaired nerve function is not known but is most likely to be due to the accumulation of some toxic metabolite which is normally excreted by the kidney. The lesion produced is a demyelination and it commonly affects the longer fibres initially. Clinically the sensory neuropathy presents little problem and it is not until late that the motor neuropathy becomes manifest as a weakness of dorsiflexion of the ankle with the associated foot-drop. The autonomic neuropathy may in part explain the occurrence of gastrointestinal motility disorders and the occasional marked postural hypotension.

Neuropathy can be quantified by motor nerve conduction velocity studies and the progression of the lesion can be followed by sequential studies. Sensory function can also be electrically tested. The involvement of the autonomic fibres can be measured by the blood pressure rise to sustained hand grip and the change in the heart rate during a Valsalva manoeuvre.

There is no satisfactory treatment of uraemic neuropathy although improvement occurs with dialysis and return to normal is known after successful transplantation.

MYOPATHY. Renal failure is frequently accompanied by generalized muscle weakness. The pathogenesis is not known but probably includes a combination of:

1. Poor nutrition.

2. Hyperparathyroidism.

3. Vitamin D deficiency.

4. Disorders of electrolyte metabolism, particularly divalent cations.

Clinically the myopathy is most noticeable in the proximal muscles and there is frequently difficulty in climbing stairs, lifting and getting up from chairs. There is no satisfactory treatment although therapy to correct vitamin D deficiency, hypocalcaemia and improve nutrition help.

ENDOCRINE MALFUNCTION. The endocrine disorders associated with chronic renal failure are complex. Generally there is depression of endocrine function and clinically the most important are:

Thyroid – biochemical hypothyroidism is common but clinical hypothyroidism is rare.

Gonads – loss of libido is very common. Mild testicular atrophy occurs and in females amenorrhoea is usual in severe failure. These features may be due to the grossly elevated prolactin concentrations which are present in patients with uraemia. Gynaecomastia may develop in males.

Adrenals – function is usually normal.

Pancreas – endocrine and exocrine function grossly normal.

Pituitary – clinically normal.

Parathyroid – hyperparathyroidism common due to low ionized calcium concentrations.

There is no satisfactory treatment for the endocrine disorders. Patients with amenorrhoea may be treated with an oral contraceptive to produce a menstrual cycle but there is no advantage in this and the blood loss is clearly undesirable. The loss of libido may respond to bromocriptine therapy.

SKIN. There are two main skin problems in the uraemic patient:

*Pruritus* is a common and distressing feature. Most commonly it affects the trunk and is aggravated by warmth. It may be severe enough to prevent sleeping. It is thought to be a manifestation of hyperparathyroidism from calcium deposition in the skin. Certainly there are documented reports of the pruritus responding dramatically to parathyroidectomy in patients with hypercalcaemia. Ultraviolet phototherapy has also been advocated but is probably of little value. Antihistamines may give symptomatic relief.

*Pigmentation* gives the patient with renal failure a characteristic appearance. It is probably due to retention of pigments normally excreted in the urine but may also be due to increased pituitary melanocyte-stimulating hormone.

CARDIOVASCULAR

1. *Hypertension* occurs in approximately 80 per cent of patients with impaired renal function. It is caused by increased activity of the renin--angiotensin system, sodium retention by intrarenal mechanisms and secondary aldosteronism, and possibly also by alterations in arteriolar muscle. In many instances it is the detection of hypertension which draws attention to impaired renal function. It is important to control blood pressure as the hypertension will cause vascular damage in the kidney, particularly in arterioles, and this will lead to a further reduction in function. Frequently this is accompanied by increased renin secretion and

so a vicious circle is established. (For management of hypertension, *see* Chapter 6.)

2. *Atherosclerosis* is significantly increased in uraemia due in part to the frequency of hypertension and in part to abnormalities of lipid and carbohydrate metabolism. There is hypertriglyceridaemia and increased very low density lipoproteins from inhibition of lipoprotein lipase. In addition there is increased triglyceride synthesis by the liver due to hyperinsulinism, increased gluconeogenesis and increased mobilization of free fatty acids. The abnormalities of carbohydrate metabolism are glucose intolerance, hyperinsulinism, elevated growth hormone concentrations and increased gluconeogenesis. The net effect of these complex metabolic changes is an increase in atheroma.

   Clinically this presents as peripheral vascular disease and coronary vascular disease. In some instances, particularly older patients, the peripheral vessels can be so extensively involved that the establishment of satisfactory vascular access is impossible. There is no satisfactory treatment but clearly the concept of feeding renal failure patients a diet high in fat and carbohydrates should be abandoned.

3. *Vascular calcification* is a manifestion of hyperparathyroidism or a complication of therapy with cholecalciferol. It is a serious consequence of a normal or high plasma calcium concentration in the presence of an elevated plasma phosphate. Clinically there may be severe peripheral vascular insufficiency with skin necrosis and loss of digits. Management of uraemic patients should be aimed at avoiding this complication by careful control of plasma calcium and plasma phosphate as once vascular calcification occurs it is virtually impossible to resolve.

4. *Subarachnoid haemorrhage* has an increased frequency due to hypertension but also due to the increased frequency of berry aneurysms in patients with polycystic renal disease.

5. *Pericarditis* is a universal finding in patients with terminal renal failure. It is of serious prognosis particularly in patients proceeding to haemodialysis as heparinization may be followed by catastrophic tamponade.

SUSCEPTIBILITY TO INFECTION. In uraemia there is a diminished cellular and humoral immunity leading to an increased susceptibility to infection. Patients are particularly prone to opportunistic infections.

Urinary tract infection is a particular hazard as the development of pyelonephritis will be accompanied by further destruction of renal tissue with consequently a further deterioration of the impaired function. There is therefore a need to monitor closely for urinary infection, not forgetting that sterile pyuria may indicate tuberculosis. All infections need to be promptly and adequately treated.

ACIDOSIS. Deterioration in renal function is accompanied by a diminution in the ability to excrete hydrogen ions. This, therefore, results in a metabolic acidosis. Biochemically this is detected as a fall in pH and a reduction in the plasma bicarbonate. In the compensated state there is hyperventilation with a consequent reduction in $pCO_2$.

In the majority of patients the acidosis is asymptomatic. If the plasma bicarbonate falls below 18 mmol/l it is advisable to consider therapy with sodium bicarbonate. However, hypertension may be induced or worsened due to the sodium load, and thus if bicarbonate is used the patient must be carefully watched for hypertension and oedema. Generally it is difficult to use bicarbonate supplements in patients with glomerular diseases whereas in pyelonephritis and cystic disease there are less problems of overload.

METASTATIC CALCIFICATION. This occurs primarily from the phosphate retention and particularly if the plasma calcium is normal or elevated. Calcium deposition is found in blood vessels, particularly in hypertensive patients, skin, dystrophic tissue such as surgical scars, periarticular tissues and rarely in tendons, falx cerebri, tentorium, and pericardium. Corneal calcification is frequent and causes intense irritiation. Initially it appears as perilimbal deposits but may extend across the cornea to produce a band keratopathy.

Clinically the presentation is with pruritus, joint stiffness, vascular disease and visual deterioration and obviously depends upon the site and extent of deposition. Treatment is difficult and management should be aimed at preventing the initial deposition occurring. This is best achieved by phosphate control and maintenance of the plasma calcium in the low normal range.

**Management.** The management of a patient with chronic renal failure can be considered as having three parts:

A. Initial baseline studies to determine the nature of the underlying disease and the extent of the severity.

B. Treatment aimed at relieving the uraemia, anaemia, osteodystrophy and any potentially reversible condition.

C. Active measures to remove waste products by either peritoneal dialysis, haemodialysis or transplantation.

A. BASELINE STUDIES

1. Careful and detailed clinical examination, paying particular attention to the cardiovascular system for hypertension, cardiomegaly, pericarditis, and peripheral vascular disease and to the genito-urinary system for renal size and the possibility of obstruction (rectal and/or vaginal examination essential).

2. Determine the nature of the underlying pathology by suitable biochemical, radiological and biopsy investigations.
3. Establish the degree of functional impairment by:
   Urinalysis.
   Blood urea, creatinine and electrolytes.
   Creatinine clearance.
   Urinary electrolyte excretion.
   Protein excretion and selectivity.
   Urinary acidification.
   Urinary concentration.
4. Document the extent of systemic complications by:
   Full blood count, including platelet count, plasma calcium and phosphate.
   Urine culture on at least three occasions, including extended culture for T.B. if sterile pyuria present.
   Skeletal survey including specific examination such as fine grain films of hands looking specifically for secondary hyperparathyroidism.
5. Specific investigations looking for possible systemic disease, e.g.
   ANF or anti-DNA antibodies.
   Hepatitis B antigen.
   Complement studies.
   Bacterial and viral antibodies.

B. TREATMENT OF AGGRAVATING FACTORS, POTENTIALLY REVERSIBLE CONDITIONS AND URAEMIA
1. Relieve any obstruction, if present.
2. Achieve correct fluid and electrolyte balance, as determined by clinical examination, daily weighing and knowledge of urine volume and composition.
3. Treat hypertension, if present (Chapter 6).
4. Treat any urinary tract infection appropriately and follow-up carefully with repeated urine cultures.
5. Introduce appropriate dietary measures:
   *Protein.* Restriction of dietary protein to 40 g daily should be instituted when the blood urea is 20 mmol/l (120 mg per cent) or the serum creatinine is 4 mmol/l (4 mg per cent), if this fails to hold the blood urea steady or produce a fall then the intake can be further reduced to 30 g daily and even 20 g daily. Intake should never be reduced below 20 g daily in the adult as this will result in loss of muscle mass due to normal catabolism.
   *Fluid.* The daily fluid intake will depend to a large extent on the nature of the underlying disease. It should be restricted to a volume equivalent to the urine output plus an allowance of 600 ml daily for insensible loss. This allowance should be increased in hot weather and if the patient is pyrexial. Generally

patients with disease of the glomeruli and cortex have low urine volumes whereas patients with medullary disease have high volumes.

*Sodium.* Restriction is required in oedematous and nephrotic patients and this is usually in the form of a 'no added salt' diet. Rarely, more stringent restriction is required. In patients with salt-losing states there may be a requirement for sodium supplements either as chloride and/or bicarbonate salts. This can be determined from a knowledge of the urinary sodium excretion obtained as part of the initial assessment.

*Potassium.* Restriction is generally required once the creatinine clearance has fallen below 20 ml/min. High potassium-containing foods should be avoided and if the potassium remains in excess of 5·5 mmol/l then exchange resins can be used (e.g. calcium resin 15 g orally b.d.). Sodium containing resins are to be avoided in view of the frequent need to restrict sodium intake.

6. Osteodystrophy and anaemia should be managed along lines indicated (*see* p. 68).

C. ACTIVE MEASURES. The measures available to remove waste products are peritoneal dialysis, haemodialysis and renal transplantation. These techniques each have advantages and disadvantages and the success of treatment depends to a large extent upon opting for the most appropriate form of therapy for any patient at a given time.

### Peritoneal Dialysis

INTRODUCTION. Peritoneal dialysis is an effective method of correcting uraemia. It is based on the fact that urea and uraemic toxins can cross the peritoneal membrane. If fluid is introduced into the peritoneal cavity it will equilibrate with the extracellular fluid and removal of the introduced fluid will therefore result in a loss from the patient of the substances which have diffused across the peritoneal membrane.

The fluid introduced into the peritoneal cavity must be sterile and have a composition, with respect to major ions, similar to that of extracellular fluid. Normally the fluid used has a composition of: sodium 140 mmol/l, calcium 1 mmol/l, chloride 100 mmol/l and magnesium 1·5 mmol/l. Potassium, in the form of potassium chloride, can be added as required. The anions are balanced by the acetate (approximately 40 mmol/l) which is metabolized in the body to bicarbonate. Isotonicity is achieved by the addition of glucose to a concentration of 1·36 per cent. If the patient is fluid overloaded then fluid may be attracted into the peritoneal cavity by the use of hypertonic dialysate. This is achieved by the addition of extra glucose to achieve a fluid concentration of 5 per cent. Commercial solutions are readily available and most suppliers provide a range of solutions suitable for the majority of needs.

INDICATIONS. Peritoneal dialysis may be used for both acute and chronic renal failure.

In acute renal failure it may be used in:

1. Patients whose blood urea is rising relatively slowly.
2. Patients who have not had abdominal surgery.
3. Severe fluid overload and/or hyperkalaemia where haemodialysis facilities are not immediately available.
4. Post cardiothoracic surgery where the cardiovascular status is unstable and thus unlikely to sustain the haemodynamic changes of haemodialysis.
5. Very small children where vascular access is difficult.
6. Elderly patients if cardiovascular problems exist.

In chronic renal failure it is of value:

1. Where haemodialysis facilities are absent or inadequate.
2. In very young patients.
3. In old patients, particularly if cardiovascular disease is present.
4. In patients with poor vascular access for haemodialysis due to previous access procedures or hypoplastic vessels.
5. In patients with diabetes mellitus.
6. In patients whose arteriovenous fistula has not matured sufficiently to permit satisfactory haemodialysis.
7. In any patient who is not progressing satisfactorily on haemodialysis.

There is thus no clear indication for peritoneal dialysis but it should be considered for all patients whose renal function has declined to the point where uraemia is becoming symptomatic.

PROCEDURE. Satisfactory peritoneal dialysis requires the insertion of a cannula into the peritoneal cavity with a free flow of fluid into and out of the cavity. Several types of cannula are available and choice depends on personal preference and the type of dialysis to be undertaken.

In the situation where only a few dialyses are to be undertaken it is common to use a relatively stiff cannula which is introduced in the midline approximately half way between the symphysis pubis and the umbilicus. Local anaesthetic is introduced into the skin and infiltrated down to the peritoneum. A small stab incision in the skin is made and the cannula with its trochar is introduced so that the tip of the cannula lies in the most dependent part of the pelvis. Once through the peritoneum the trochar is withdrawn slightly to prevent the puncture of bowel or bladder. It is essential to ensure that the patient has an empty bladder before commencing the procedure. The cannula is attached to the skin by elastoplast tape after a suitable small dressing has been applied round the entry site. The cannula can then be connected by a suitable line and three-way tap to the bags containing the dialysate and a suitable drainage bag.

The dialysate fluid requires to be warmed prior to installation or hypothermia may result. It takes approximately 10 min to run 2 l of fluid into the peritoneal cavity and it is left to equilibrate for 20 min. Drainage takes 20 min and thus each cycle lasts for 1 hour. In this way some 48 l are used in a 24 h period and this will result in the blood urea falling by approximately one-half. Most dialyses will last for about 30–36 h. They are then repeated as dictated by the patient's clinical and biochemical status.

In some instances pain is experienced, particularly if hypertonic solution is used. This can be overcome by the addition of a small amount of local anaesthetic to the dialysate. Similarly in some patients there is considerable difficulty with fibrin clots forming in the cannula and this can be overcome by the addition of 600 u of heparin to the 2 l of dialysate. In the first few exchanges it is common to have some slight bloodstaining but this usually resolves satisfactorily. If it persists or is heavy it raises the possibility of vessel perforation and this requires immediate attention. Only very rarely will surgical intervention be required.

In circumstances where repeated or continued dialyses are to be performed then the use of a 'soft' cannula is advisable. This can be inserted with a specially designed introducer or by direct vision. The cannula is frequently sited lateral to the midline and it passes through a subcutaneous tunnel to enter through the peritoneum a short distance from the site of skin insertion.

Dialysis can be performed for a fixed period of time and then the cannula closed off with a spigot until the next session. This is complicated by a high incidence of infection and so a preferable method is to exchange fluid continuously. In this way 2 l of fluid are introduced into the peritoneal cavity and left for 4 hours with the patient fully mobile. At the end of this time the fluid is drained out and replaced. Five 2 l exchanges are therefore undertaken each day and the patient can very quickly be taught to perform this himself at home. This technique, continuous ambulatory peritoneal dialysis, provides an alternative to haemodialysis for certain patients.

## ADVANTAGES OF PERITONEAL DIALYSIS

1. Efficient removal of uraemic toxins with the added advantage that the range of substances removed is greater than by haemodialysis.
2. There are no sudden swings of blood chemistry and so removal of fluid and waste products is not associated with disequilibration or hypotension.
3. The technique is easy to perform and requires no expensive machinery.
4. In continuous ambulatory peritoneal dialysis there is stable blood

chemistry and as removal of waste products is continuous it can
be said to be more 'physiological'.

DISADVANTAGES OF PERITONEAL DIALYSIS

1. The introduction of the cannula may produce perforation of
   bowel, bladder or blood vessel. The perforation of a major blood
   vessel may be associated with catastrophic haemorrhage and the
   cannula should only be removed under surgical control. Perforation of bladder or bowel rarely produces any major problem.
2. Infection is common especially if a careful sterile technique has
   not been used. Most infection is introduced through the skin
   incision and it can be extremely troublesome. It is advisable
   to monitor every second dialysis exchange by culture so that if
   an infection arises appropriate antibiotic therapy can be used.
   Antibiotics can be added to the dialysis fluid but this is not
   recommended as a routine.
3. The instillation of 2 l of fluid into the peritoneal cavity results
   in the elevation of the diaphragm and thus may lead to hypostatic pneumonia. This is particularly the case when the hard
   cannula is employed as patients are frequently immobile
   during the procedure. Fluid may also pass from the peritoneal
   to the pleural cavity and thus may cause further respiratory
   embarrassment.
4. Ileus may occur, particularly if infection develops.
5. Clotting may occur in the cannula but this is usually rapidly
   corrected by the addition of heparin.
6. Patients who subsequently transfer to haemodialysis seem to
   have an increased incidence of ascites.
7. In continuous ambulatory peritoneal dialysis there may be the
   appearance of an accelerated atherosclerosis. The mechanism of
   this is not certain but may be related to the carbohydrate load
   which results from the dialysate glucose.

   There are thus advantages and disadvantages of this procedure.
In a patient the decision to use peritoneal dialysis can only be
made after carefully considering these factors. In most cases the
advantages outweigh the disadvantages, and the incidence of serious
complications is low.


**Haemodialysis**

INTRODUCTION. Haemodialysis is a method of removing substances
from the blood by employing a semipermeable membrane. The
technique of dialysis has been used by industry for many years but
it was not until the pioneering work of Willem Kolff in the 1940s
that it became applied to the removal of uraemic toxins from blood.
Facilities for undertaking this technique were not generally available
prior to 1960 but since then there has been a rapid expansion and

haemodialysis is now widely available for the treatment of acute and chronic renal failure.

PRINCIPLES. Haemodialysis is based on the fact that many of the substances which have been suggested as the cause of uraemia are of small size and capable of diffusing through membranes of specific characteristics. The membranes used for haemodialysis are readily permeable to low molecular weight substances but are impermeable to substances of a high molecular weight, i.e. those of a molecular weight in excess of 1000. The fact that haemodialysis keeps patients with chronic renal failure reasonably well is remarkable when one considers that we do not know the cause of uraemia nor the nature of the materials removed during haemodialysis. It has been suggested that many of the features of uraemia are caused by middle molecules and these are only poorly removed by current haemodialysis techniques, so clearly there is scope for improvement in membrane technology.

Haemodialysis membranes are relatively unselective regarding the material which passes through them. Waste products such as urea and creatinine are readily permeable as are amino acids, water-soluble vitamins and sugars. It is uncertain whether the complications of long-term haemodialysis are due to the poor removal of high molecular weight toxic factors or the excessive removal and subsequent depletion of low molecular weight essential nutrients.

The semipermeable membrane separates the patient's blood from a dialysate solution. Most current apparatus employs a 'single pass' system where the patient's blood flows across the membrane while the dialysate flows on the other side of the membrane in the opposite direction. Substances can cross the membrane in both directions and so the composition of the dialysate must be carefully controlled and usually contains sodium 140 mmol/l, calcium 1·5 mmol/l, magnesium 1·0 mmol/l, chloride 100 mmol/l and acetate 40 mmol/l. The acetate is metabolized in the body to bicarbonate. Most dialysate is now devoid of glucose. Fluid can be made to cross the membrane by increasing the hydrostatic pressure in the blood compartment and/or applying a negative pressure to the dialysate compartment.

INDICATIONS. Haemodialysis can be used for acute and chronic renal failure.

1. In acute renal failure haemodialysis is of particular value for those patients whose blood urea is rising rapidly and who would not achieve satisfactory biochemical control using peritoneal dialysis. It is also of value where recent abdominal surgery makes peritoneal dialysis undesirable.

2. In chronic renal failure where the decision is to offer replacement therapy, it is always advisable to have a period of haemodialysis prior to transplantation as the patient is physically improved.

The correct time to commence a patient on regular haemodialysis is difficult to determine but it is advisable as soon as the patient develops symptoms of uraemia (anorexia, pericarditis, pulmonary oedema, electrolyte disorders not controlled adequately by diet, neuropathy).

HAEMODIALYSIS TECHNIQUES. Since the introduction of haemodialysis there have been many changes and improvements in the techniques employed but the basic principles remain unchanged. During a haemodialysis session blood is continuously removed and passed through a device wherein a semipermeable membrane separates the blood from the dialysis solution (dialysate). This device, the artificial kidney, comprises a compartment through which the blood flows, a compartment through which dialysate flows and a supporting framework so that the internal structure, particularly the blood film thickness, is kept fairly constant.

The initial design consisted of a double layer of membrane wound around a drum which rotated in a bath of dialysate. This was an efficient but rather cumbersome device. Later developments produced an artificial kidney which was made from membranes supported by polypropylene boards thus greatly reducing the size and providing a means of easily renewing the membrane after each dialysis session. This kidney became widely used and with minor modification is still popular. Two other types of artificial kidney are available and are in regular use. The first is the coil-type kidney where a tube of dialysis membrane is wound around a plastic supporting meshwork and the second is where the membrane has been spun into very fine hollow fibres which are then packed into a plastic cylinder to form the capillary kidney. The performances of these kidneys varies considerably but is dependent on the surface area of the membrane together with the degree of turbulence produced in the blood compartment, the thickness of the membrane and the membrane material. Current developments involve mainly improvements to the membrane so that more selective dialysis can be undertaken.

In the early stage of dialysis design the artificial kidney was rotated in a large bath of dialysate. The first improvement was to provide a pump which forced the dialysate through the kidney thereby overcoming the difficult problem of coupling static blood lines to a rotating artificial kidney. The next major development was the introduction of proportioning pumps which would take suitable treated water and a concentrated salt solution to produce dialysate of a determined composition. This abolished the need to provide large tanks of dialysate and so greatly reduced the bulk of the apparatus. More recently the Redy system has been introduced where a small volume of dialysate can be constantly regenerated by using columns which will absorb waste products and which will trap urea after its conversion to ammonia by the action of urease. Once again this has greatly reduced the bulk of the apparatus but has considerably increased the cost due to the need for the additional absorbing column. Development continues and it is highly likely that the trend towards more efficient dialysers and miniaturization will continue.

The blood removed during dialysis requires to be heparinized to prevent clotting. This can be achieved by giving a dose of heparin at the beginning of a dialysis session and then giving regular bolus injections or a continuous infusion over the dialysis session. If the heparin is stopped approximately 1 hour before the end of treatment then there is seldom any need for reversal with protamine. In certain circumstances such as after surgery or in the presence of pericarditis it is advisable to avoid systemic heparinization. In such situations dialysis can be achieved by regional heparinization where heparin is continuously infused to the blood coming from the patient while, simultaneously, protamine is added to the blood returning to the patient. This allows for satisfactory heparinization of the blood in the dialyser while maintaining the patient with a satisfactory intact clotting mechanism.

VASCULAR ACCESS. Satisfactory vascular access is an essential requirement for haemodialysis. Three main methods are currently available.

1. *Quinton–Scribner Shunt.* Regular haemodialysis for chronic renal failure did not become widely available until the development of the shunt. This device consists of a small hollow piece of Teflon to which is attached a length of Silastic tubing. This is inserted in a suitable artery and a similar inserted in a suitable vein. The two are then connected together so that the blood flowing down the artery passes through the Silastic to the vein. During dialysis the two pieces of Silastic are separated, thus providing an outflow to the machine and a return to the patient.

   The disadvantages of this system are:

   a. *Clotting episodes.* These can be troublesome, particularly if there is any malalignment of the vessel tip and the vessel or if there has been any intimal damage during insertion. The frequency of clotting can be reduced by the use of antiplatelet drugs such as aspirin or dipyridamole or anti-coagulation with warfarin.

   b. *Infection.* The foreign material passes through the skin and thus provides a portal of entry for organisms. Once infection gains access it can be particularly difficult to eradicate.

   c. *Extrusion.* If sufficient care has not been taken to provide a satisfactory covering of skin and subcutaneous fat overlying the Silastic there may be ulceration and eventual extrusion of the device.

d. *Limitation of activity.* Due to the presence of the shunt certain sporting activities such as swimming are impossible. Bathing can prove difficult particularly if a leg shunt is present.

e. *Restricted use.* The length of time that a shunt can be used is restricted. On average a leg shunt can be used for 9–12 months and an arm shunt for 15–24 months. Thus with time it is possible to run out of suitable shunt sites. Failure is usually due to a combination of clotting and infection.

f. *Vascular insufficiency.* The insertion of a shunt occludes the vessel distally. This can result in peripheral vascular insufficiency which may not become apparent for several years.

The Teflon–Silastic shunt, although providing satisfactory vascular access, has many problems. Its use is now restricted to those patients who require urgent dialysis and therefore cannot wait for a fistula to mature and for young children who find it difficult to accept the needling of a fistula.

2. *Cimino–Brescia Fistula.* This is a system where a vein is anastomosed to an artery so that arterial blood enters the venous system producing dilatation. The distended veins are easy to puncture with a large needle and by this means blood can be removed and returned during dialysis. At the end of the procedure the needles are removed and thus no foreign material permanently enters through the skin. The patient is therefore not at risk from infection and clotting and is free from the limitations imposed by a shunt. The fistula is not entirely free from complications.

a. *Inadequate dilatation of forearm veins.* This may occur due to the small calibre of the vessels or because the vessels have been damaged from previous vascular access procedures or intravenous infusions. Females frequently have small poorly distensible veins.

b. *Increase in cardiac output.* The formation of an arteriovenous fistula may produce cardiac failure because of the necessary associated increased cardiac output. Fortunately for a fistula inserted at the wrist the flow is unlikely to be sufficient to produce this complication.

c. *Distal venous stasis.* As arterial blood enters the venous system there is a local increase in venous pressure which may cause distal venous stasis and even lead to skin necrosis.

d. *Thrombosis.* Thrombosis of the fistula is uncommon once it has become established although it may occur after surgery or any other procedure causing increased coagulation.

Fistulae provide very satisfactory vascular access but they require time for satisfactory development and should thus be inserted prior to dialysis becoming essential. In this way the patient coming to dialysis can have a good site for vascular access and therefore be established with ease on haemodialysis.

3. *Arteriovenous Grafts.* In patients with poor venous systems or multiple previous vascular access procedures it may be impossible to establish a satisfactory fistula or shunt. For these patients a synthetic graft can be placed subcutaneously joining a suitable artery with a vein. The most satisfactory results are obtained by joining the femoral artery below the inguinal ligament with a long straight synthetic graft to the long saphenous vein above the knee. A wide variety of materials are available, expanded poly-tetrafluoroethylene, Dacron velour, autogenous saphenous vein, human umbilical cord vein and bovine carotid artery, the choice depending to a large extent on the preference and experience of the surgeon undertaking the procedure.

Grafts are associated with a number of problems – clotting, infection, aneurysm formation and increasing cardiac output – but they provide a useful alternative for the patient who has vascular access problems.

MEDICAL PROBLEMS OF PATIENTS ON HAEMODIALYSIS. There are many medical problems of patients on long-term haemodialysis. These problems may be directly related to the dialysis procedure, others are due to complications of uraemia which are not corrected or only partially corrected by haemodialysis while others are due directly to the effects of long-term dialysis. An artificial kidney is a simple device which cannot be expected to assume the complex excretory and metabolic functions of the kidney and thus it must not be assumed that the use of an artificial kidney can correct completely all the multiple metabolic abnormalities of uraemia. It is remarkable that so many patients survive and are well for years on thrice or twice weekly haemodialysis.

1. *Problems associated with the Dialysis Procedure*
    a. *Disequilibrium.* This is rare but is due to the rapid lowering of blood urea. The c.s.f. equilibrates slowly and thus if the extracellular fluid urea concentration falls rapidly there will be a relative hypertonicity of the c.s.f. with the subsequent attraction of fluid through the blood/brain barrier with the development of cerebral oedema. This can be severe enough to produce headaches, fits and even respiratory arrest. It occurs most commonly during initial dialyses where the blood urea is grossly elevated. It is overcome by undertaking a very short first dialysis and gradually increasing dialysis time as the blood urea concentration comes under control.

  b. *Hypotension.* This is a common occurrence during dialysis. The cause is multifactorial. It is due to a combination of excessive fluid removal resulting in hypovolaemia, a reduction in extracellular fluid osmolality with a subsequent shift of fluid to the intracellular compartment and possibly even an autonomic neuropathy which prevents the adequate haemodynamic correction to hypovolaemia. It can be overcome by the isotonic removal of fluid in sequential haemofiltration-haemodialysis or by the infusion of saline to correct the hypovolaemia. Haemofiltration is a technique whereby fluid is removed by hydrostatic pressure alone prior to haemodialysis. In such a procedure there is the loss of isotonic fluid and so there are no shifts between the extra- and intracellular fluid.

  c. *Cramp.* This can be particularly troublesome, particularly if a low sodium dialysate is used. It is probably due to ionic shifts across muscles, and can be reduced in intensity and frequency by using a dialysate sodium of 140–144 mmol/l.

  d. *Pyrogenic reactions.* Pyrogens can cross the dialysis membrane and give reactions which consist of pyrexia, shivering, minor muscle ache and a feeling of cold. It usually signifies bacterial contamination of the water softener or some fault in the preparation of dialysis equipment.

  e. *Acetate intolerance.* Acetate forms a major anion in most dialysate solutions. It is metabolized in the body to bicarbonate but this is a rate-dependent step. The transfer of acetate from dialysate to blood may exceed the rate of metabolism, particularly when large surface area dialysers are used. The symptoms consist of nausea, vomiting, cramp and hypotension. These are, however, not specific for acetate intolerance but when present in a few patients in a unit, particularly if the patients are small and using large dialysers, should raise the possibility.

  f. *Fluid overload.* This is not truly a complication of the dialysis procedure but it arises because dialysis is intermittent and so the patient spends much of the week in the position of being unable to excrete fluid. Many patients experience intense thirst and find it difficult to adhere to their designated fluid allowance.

2. *Problems of Uraemia uncorrected by Haemodialysis*
  a. *Anaemia.* Following the commencement of haemodialysis there is frequently an increase in haematocrit but it is rare for this to return to normal. Most patients on haemodialysis have a haemoglobin of 6–9 g/dl. There is an inevitable small blood loss during each dialysis session and this contributes to

the factors already described as being responsible for uraemic anaemia (*see* p. 66). Haemodialysis not only removes some of the uraemic factors but also usually allows for a better diet and this is probably responsible for the slight improvement. Oral iron should be used regularly. It is advisable to restrict blood transfusion to a minimum.

b. *Bone disease.* Vitamin D metabolism remains deranged due to inadequate hydroxylation of cholecalciferol from 1α-hydroxylase deficiency. The osteomalacia persists and may progress, and hyperparathyroidism may also appear or progress. In addition there is evidence that aluminium accumulation may occur in bones and lead to a very resistant form of osteomalacia. The aluminium arises either from the phosphate-binding drugs such as aluminium hydroxide and/or aluminium which occurs in the water supply used for dialysis. Thus bone disease is not improved and may even become symptomatic during dialysis. It can be helped by the administration of one alpha to keep the plasma calcium in the normal range to prevent hyperparathyroidism developing, the restriction of phosphate-binding drugs to a minimum and the use of de-ionized or reverse osmosis treated water for the manufacture of dialysate.

c. *Infection.* The increased susceptibility of the uraemic patient to infection is not corrected by dialysis.

d. *Hypertension.* In many patients with good dialysis and adequate control of sodium and fluid intake there is resolution or considerable improvement in blood pressure control. In a number of patients, however, there are continuing problems and bilateral nephrectomy may be required. This procedure is not without hazard and may only be followed by a reduced requirement of hypotensive drugs. This presumably is due to irreversible vascular changes consequent on longstanding hypertension.

e. *Calcium metabolism.* Calcium malabsorption continues and this may result in hypocalcaemia and subsequent hyperparathyroidism. It is best controlled by using a dialysate with a calcium concentration of 1·5 mmol/l and a dose of one alpha sufficient to maintain the pre-dialysis calcium in the normal range.

f. *Gonadal dysfunction.* Amenorrhoea and loss of libido are uncorrected by dialysis. This may be due to the continuing high prolactin concentrations. This may be improved by the use of bromocriptine.

3. *Complications of Long-term Haemodialysis*
   a. *Vascular disease.* This is due to the increased incidence of

*atheroma* as a result of hyperlipidaemia, hypertension and the carbohydrate load from dialysate glucose. In addition, many patients, particularly those who have been on dialysis for many years, will have had *vascular access procedures* with a reduction in peripheral blood flow. To this can be added the *metastatic calcification* which occurs in the vessels of some patients as a result of the elevated plasma phosphate. Vascular disease is very variable but its incidence increases with age and length of time on dialysis. Prevention is difficult but the effects can be minimized by avoiding shunts, controlling hypertension, controlling hyperlipidaemia and avoiding hyperphosphataemia.

b. *Cardiomyopathy.* This is observed in a small number of patients and consists of a grossly enlarged heart with poor myocardial function and dilated left ventricle. It may occur due to prolonged hypertension or coronary vascular disease. It should not be due to nutritional deficiency but unsuspected alcoholism may occur. In a number of patients no cause can be found and so it is presumed to be due to some unidentified factor related to dialysis. Treatment is extremely difficult but control of blood pressure and stringent avoidance of fluid overload is mandatory.

c. *Psychological disorders.* The incidence of minor psychological disturbances, anxiety and depression, is high and is probably related to the patient's dependency for survival on a machine. Major disturbances are rare although suicide probably has a higher incidence than recognized. The lack of major problems may be related to selection procedures.

d. *Hypersplenism.* This occurs in 1–2 per cent of dialysis patients and may require splenectomy. It adds to the problem of anaemia and should be considered in any patient with profound anaemia, particularly if requiring repeated blood transfusions.

e. *Dementia.* Dialysis dementia or progressive dialysis encephalopathy is a well-recognized syndrome consisting initially of mild speech disorder, stuttering, periodic speech arrest and anomia progressing to epileptiform convulsions, myoclonus and dysphagia. The speech disorder becomes more severe until mutism develops. The majority of patients die from bronchopneumonia as a result of inhalation from dysphagia. The cause is thought to be aluminium intoxication from the aluminium contained in dialysis water supplies and phosphate-binding agents. It can be prevented by the avoidance of aluminium but once it appears it only rarely improves in spite of all measures. It would appear virtually impossible to remove accumulated aluminium.

    *f. Metastatic calcification.* Plasma phosphate concentrations remain elevated in spite of adequate dialysis. If the plasma calcium is elevated either due to one alpha or a high dialysate calcium then metastatic calcification will occur. It is most common in skin producing pruritus; in eyes giving perilimbal calcification and in severe cases a band keratopathy; in vessels giving hypertension and vascular insufficiency; and in periarticular tissue presumably due to minor trauma. It is best avoided by careful control of the plasma phosphate and strict avoidance of hypercalcaemia.

RESPONSE OF URAEMIA TO DIALYSIS. Haemodialysis corrects some of the features of uraemia but does not replace all the functions of the kidney. The excretory function can be replaced in a non-selective way while the endocrine and metabolic malfunctions persist unchanged.

*Uraemic Symptoms.* These are improved, particularly the anorexia and nausea, although weakness and lack of energy may persist. Generally within 6 weeks of commencing haemodialysis the patient notices considerable symptomatic improvement.

*Anaemia.* Haematocrit rises slightly but anaemia persists.

*Osteodystrophy.* No marked change as the abnormalities of vitamin D metabolism persist. The hyperparathyroid element of the osteodystrophy can be considerably reduced by maintaining a satisfactory plasma calcium with a correct dialysate calcium and one alpha. The osteomalacia may become more severe due to the added problem of aluminium and other trace element accumulation.

*Neuropathy.* Both motor and sensory neuropathy improve with adequate dialysis. Motor nerve conduction velocities can be used as an index of adequacy of dialysis. A return to normal may occur. Autonomic nerve function also improves although a return to normal has not been documented.

*Myopathy.* Muscle power generally improves with adequate dialysis.

*Endocrine Malfunction.* Little or no response to dialysis. Most of the abnormalities persist and some, such as libido, may deteriorate.

*Skin.* Pruritus is common in dialysis patients and is frequently associated with disorders of calcium metabolism. Pigmentation is generally unchanged by conventional dialysis and may even deepen in some patients.

*Cardiovascular.* Hypertension is usually more easily controlled following the institution of dialysis. With good dialysis control of weight, fluid and sodium intake it is normally possible to reduce and sometimes stop hypotensive therapy. Some patients, in spite of all measures, continue with severe hypertension and bilateral nephrectomy should be considered if the patient requires more than three hypotensive drugs or experiences unacceptable side effects from therapy. Atherosclerosis usually is unchanged by dialysis but in a significant number of patients becomes more severe and, in addition, may be aggravated by increased calcification. Patients managed by continuous ambulatory peritoneal dialysis have experienced, in some instances, an accelerated atherosclerosis. Pericarditis is virtually a universal finding in patients with chronic renal failure severe enough to warrant replacement therapy. This responds well to dialysis and usually resolves within the first 4–6 weeks of treatment. Pericarditis appearing after this time is either an indication of inadequate dialysis or the development of some other form such as viral pericarditis.

*Infection.* Although there is an improvement in reticulo-endothelial function there is still impaired resistance to infections.

*Acidosis.* Dialysate contains acetate which is metabolized to bicarbonate. The acidosis of chronic renal failure therefore resolves when dialysis is conducted efficiently and regularly. The pre-dialysis plasma bicarbonate should be in excess of 18 mmol/l and preferably above 20 mmol/l. There are considerable problems associated with the use of a bicarbonate dialysate but the development of more efficient apparatus will overcome this problem and it is likely that acetate will be replaced by bicarbonate thus producing a more physiological dialysis as well as avoiding the problems of acetate intolerance.

*Metastatic Calcifications.* This problem may resolve on dialysis if the plasma phosphate concentration is carefully controlled. In some patients, even with large doses of phosphate-binding agents, it is not possible to achieve a satisfactory plasma phosphate concentration and so metastatic calcification may progress, particularly if a high dialysate calcium concentration is used.

PROGNOSIS. The survival of patients on haemodialysis depends on many factors:

1. The underlying nature of the renal failure – patients with systemic disease have a poorer prognosis compared with those with glomerulonephritis or pyelonephritis.
2. The age at onset of dialysis – generally older patients have a poorer prognosis due to the increased incidence of ischaemic heart disease.
3. The duration of uraemia prior to the institution of haemodialysis – the longer the time the greater the incidence of uraemic complications and consequently the poorer the prognosis.

4. The effectiveness of dialysis and drugs in controlling hypertension.
5. The degree to which a given patient adheres to the fluid and dietary restrictions – excessive interdialytic weight gain is associated with a poor prognosis.
6. The adequacy of the dialysis procedure to control uraemia.

Thus the prognosis depends on many factors other than the efficiency of treatment and patient compliance. Home dialysis patients have a 5-year survival of approximately 80 per cent. Hospital dialysis patients have a 5-year survival of approximately 65 per cent. The difference in these survival figures can be accounted for by patient selection and the fact that the patient on home dialysis is better rehabilitated.

The major causes of death in dialysis patients are: ischaemic heart disease, infections, cerebrovascular disease and malignancy. The increased death rate from vascular disease is due to the increased incidence of atheroma and hypertension. The increased incidence of infections and malignancy is probably due to suppression of the reticulo-endothelial system.

Survival on dialysis is improving due to improved dialyser design, improved membranes and a reduction in dietary manoeuvres as a consequence of improved dialysis.

SELECTION OF PATIENTS. In the past considerable emphasis was placed on the selection of patients for dialysis. This was due to the fact that this technique was in its infancy and there was a very considerable shortage of machines. In such circumstances there was a need to select patients for haemodialysis carefully so that the limited facilities were put to maximum use. Fortunately the availability of dialysis has markedly improved and now there is no need to select patients due to lack of resources.

There are, however, certain factors which should be taken into account.
1. Age, at the lower end age is not considered a contraindication but it is difficult to undertake regular haemodialysis in a patient of less than 15 kg weight. At the upper end the incidence of cardiovascular disease increases with age and patients in excess of 65 years may have considerable problems with respect to vascular access and cardiac stability.
2. Systemic disease; patients who have renal failure as part of a widespread systemic disease are unlikely to benefit from dialysis as their systemic disease is likely to give progressive multisystem failure. In diabetes mellitus the patient with severe retinopathy, severe peripheral vascular disease and neuropathy is unlikely to benefit from dialysis while another patient with diabetes mellitus and only minor complications will progress satisfactorily.

Fortunately in the vast majority of patients there is no doubt about the advisability of dialysis. All patients who can expect an improvement in the quality of their life should be treated.

HOSPITAL, SATELLITE OR HOME DIALYSIS? It is possible to perform haemodialysis in hospital units, satellite or limited-care units or at home.

Hospital dialysis has attractions as far as the patient is concerned. There is staff to prepare the machine and clear away after treatment. There is no disruption to his home and little to his family. There is a reduction in stress as trained staff are always at hand to deal with any problem. The disadvantages are the travelling time to and from hospital and the fact that dialysis times will be dictated by the hospital unit. The major disadvantage, however, comes from the fact that each unit will only be able to support a finite number of patients and new patients will only be able to be accepted following removal of an existing patient by transplantation or death. Assuming each patient receives treatment for 4 hours thrice weekly then the maximum number of patients a given unit can support will be six times the number of dialysis spaces.

Satellite, limited-care or hostel dialysis offers a facility which is some way between hospital and home dialysis. Such units can be established near to the patient's home and thus reduce travelling time. They require minimum staffing as many patients are trained to undertake the majority of procedures unaided. They are cheaper to run than a hospital unit and they avoid the cost of single home units. The disadvantage is the continued need for travel, the restriction of dialysis times and the finite number of patients accommodated. Home dialysis has the advantage that the patient is free from travel and may choose his dialysis time to suit his own and his family's convenience. This allows him a greater chance of full rehabilitation as he will be free to undertake a normal week's work and dialyse in the evening. The disadvantage is the cost of installation and supply and the fact that the equipment is only used by one person for a relatively short time in the week.

There is no best form of dialysis. The choice between hospital, satellite or home depends on geography, finances, presence of help at home and the ability to train the patient. The most satisfactory solution is to have the three forms available and to choose the most adequate for each given patient.

HEPATITIS. Outbreaks of hepatitis have occurred in the patients and staff of many dialysis units. In the majority of instances this has been due to serum hepatitis which is due to the hepatitis B virus (Australia antigen). It is transmitted by blood, serum, blood products and body secretions such as tears, saliva and semen. It gains access through breaks in the skin, from piercing the skin with an infected needle and possibly through mucous membranes. It can be transmitted by blood or blood product transfusion. The virulence of the virus is variable but there has been a significant mortality among patients and staff and this has led to stringent precautions to avoid the introduction of the virus into units. The precautions which have been most successful are:

1. The screening of all blood to be transfused for the presence of hepatitis B antigen and the restriction of all transfusions to a minimum.
2. The avoidance of the use of any blood product which is not guaranteed free from virus. Albumin and PPF are safe as they are pasteurized during preparation whereas fibrinogen and coagulation factors are not safe.
3. The total prohibition of eating or smoking in dialysis areas by staff.
4. The regular screening of patients and staff for hepatitis B virus. Patients becoming positive must be segregated and dialysed in a separate unit. Staff must not return to work until they are negative to antigen testing and preferably only after they have become antibody positive.
5. Reduction in blood sampling to a minimum compatible with good patient management.
6. The careful disposal of all sharp objects such as needles in an attempt to avoid staff accidentally piercing skin.

### Transplantation

INTRODUCTION. The transplantation of a normal kidney to a patient with chronic renal failure is now an established technique. In the past twenty years it has become more common and the numbers of patients being transplanted continues to rise year by year.

There are two major problems in transplantation – the handling of the donor kidney and the control of the rejection process. The first of these problems has been largely solved. Cadaver kidneys are now obtained with as short a warm ischaemia as possible and then they are rapidly cooled by perfusion. It is now possible to store these organs for up to 20 h which allows them to be transported a considerable distance if necessary and also allows for some pre-treatment of the potential recipient. The second problem, however, remains the most difficult aspect of transplantation. Considerable advances in immunosuppression have been made in the past twenty years but there is a significant number of kidneys lost due to rejection. This will only improve by improved recipient selection and improved immunosuppressive drugs.

PRINCIPLES OF TRANSPLANTATION. The success of transplantation depends upon careful donor and recipient selection. Kidneys may be obtained from living relations or from cadavers.

Live related donors are either identical twins, parents or siblings. In the identical twin situation no immunosuppression is required and so the recipient is freed from all the complications of anti-rejection therapy. In non-identical twins and other relatives immunosuppression is still required although the dose of drugs required may be less than in a cadaver transplant. Before accepting a relative as a donor it is necessary to satisfy the following criteria:

1. The donor and recipient must be ABO compatible.
2. The donor must have two normal kidneys and a normal urinary tract as demonstrated by i.v.p. and arteriogram.
3. The donor, recipient and their respective families must be agreeable to the transplant operation.
4. The donor should be at no risk of developing the same renal disease as the recipient.

Normally the investigation of a potential living donor includes:

1. Full blood count, urea and electrolytes.
2. Blood grouping and tissue typing.
3. Urinalysis and culture.
4. Intravenous pyelogram.
5. Creatinine clearance and protein excretion.
6. Arteriogram.
7. Mixed lymphocyte culture between donor and recipient.
8. Determination of the cytomegalovirus status of the donor and recipient. (It is inadvisable to transplant a kidney from a donor who is known to have or have had cytomegalovirus infection to a recipient who has never had the infection. Such transfers are associated with an increased risk of rejection.)

Cadaver kidneys are obtained from patients who die from such conditions as trauma, subarachnoid haemorrhage or primary cerebral tumours. The donor must be free from infection and have normally functioning kidneys up to the time of death.

The recipient of a kidney must:

1. Be ABO compatible with the donor.
2. Have a normal lower urinary tract.
3. Be free from infection, particularly urinary tract infection.
4. Be rehabilitated by dialysis.
5. Have blood pressure adequately controlled.
6. Be willing to have a transplant operation.

IMMUNOSUPPRESSION. In the identical twin situation no immunosuppression is required. For all other patients rejection is controlled by:

1. *Prednisolone.* Starting with a daily dose of 100 mg and reducing to 30 mg daily by 30 days. Thereafter the dose is reduced by

2·5 mg decrements until a maintenance dose of 15 mg daily is reached some 6 months post-transplant. After a year it should be possible to reduce to 10 mg daily but this requires careful monitoring.

2. *Azathioprine.* Commenced at day 1 in a dose of 2 mg/kg, i.e. 150 mg daily for the average adult. This dose is continued but adjusted as required, depending on the white cell and platelet counts. Azathioprine is continued indefinitely at 2 mg/kg.

3. *Cyclophosphamide.* This is a useful alternative to azathioprine and may be used in patients who are sensitive to azathioprine.

4. *Methylprednisolone.* This is used for acute rejection episodes and is given 1 g i.v. on three consecutive days. This may be repeated as required but it is inadvisable to give more than 15 g to any individual patient.

5. *Antilymphocytic Globulin (ALG).* This has been used in the immediate post-transplant period and for the treatment of acute rejection.

6. *Graft Irradiation.* This is no longer standard practice.

To avoid undue complications of immunosuppressive therapy it is necessary to monitor all patients carefully. This requires daily observations initially with gradually increasing intervals as the graft becomes settled. The aim of immunosuppression is to control the rejection process with the minimum of therapy.

RESPONSE OF URAEMIA TO TRANSPLANTATION. The restoration of renal function by a transplanted kidney is accompanied by a rapid resolution of the manifestation of uraema. Symptomatically the patients are much improved but this is also in part due to the elation at being free from dialysis and the effect of the steroids. Anaemia responds briskly and a reticulocyte response is one of the early indications of success. Vitamin D metabolism is rapidly restored to normal although this may be masked by steroids in the first few months. Many of the problems of uraemia and dialysis are satisfactorily resolved but replaced by complications of the necessary immunosuppressive therapy.

COMPLICATIONS OF TRANSPLANTATION. There are many problems, medical and surgical, which can arise in the transplanted patient and it is best to consider them in relation to the time from transplantation.

1. *Immediate*

a. *Anaesthesia.* This requires care and experience as the patient will be anaemic, will have disordered drug metabolism and will not tolerate much in the way of i.v. fluids.

b. *Rejection.* If preformed antibodies are present a hyperacute rejection will occur which will become obvious shortly after vascular flow is established. The kidney swells and becomes very dark. It must be removed. This problem should not occur if adequate direct cross-match between donor and recipient has been performed.

c. *Electrolyte disorders.* Starvation preoperatively together with prolonged anaesthesia and possible transfusion make hyperkalaemia common. This will be compounded if there is any inadequate ventilation postoperatively. The serum potassium must be carefully monitored after the surgery.

d. *Fluid overload.* In many instances there is a variable period of delayed renal function and so considerable care has to be taken during surgery and until function is adequately established to avoid fluid overload.

e. *Bleeding.* This may present a problem, particularly if dialysis was performed immediately prior to surgery.

2. *Postoperative Problems*

a. *Acute tubular necrosis.* A significant number of transplanted kidneys do not have primary function. The delay in the onset of function is very variable. A number will have satisfactory function within 3–5 days and it is unlikely that this short delay is due to tubular necrosis. However, a number take from 2 to 3 weeks to recover and it is possible in these patients that the donor organ experienced an insult sufficient to produce a tubular necrosis. It is frequently difficult to differentiate between delayed onset of function and rejection and renal biopsy may be of help in such circumstances.

b. *Rejection.* This is most likely to appear between the 10th and 14th day. It is characterized by a fall in urine output accompanied by a rise in plasma creatinine and urea. Frequently there is a mild pyrexia and the patient may complain of flu-like symptoms.

   On examination the kidney is enlarged. It is treated by bolus i.v. infusions of 1 g methylprednisolone for 3 consecutive days. The prednisolone and azathioprine dosage is usually left unchanged. Most rejection episodes can be overcome by this regimen but many patients experience repeated episodes.

c. *Steroid therapy.* In the first month after transplantation the patient receives a fairly high dose of steroids and may therefore develop *steroid psychosis* and/or *steroid-induced diabetes mellitus.* A careful watch needs to be kept for glycosuria, particularly if polyuria develops.

d. *Immunosuppressive therapy.* Patients vary in their susceptibility to azathioprine and so in the first month after transplantation the white blood cell and platelet count require daily monitoring. Leucopenia and thrombocytopenia are not uncommon and are best treated by a suitable reduction in the azathioprine dose.

e. *Infection.* In the initial stages of immunosuppression there is an impaired resistance to infection and this requires careful nursing and constant monitoring.

f. *Venous thrombosis.* Deep vein thrombosis is most common in the leg on the same side as the transplant. This is presumably due to alteration to blood flow in the iliac vein consequent upon the anastomosis of the renal vein. In many instances there is mild swelling of the leg with no evidence of venous thrombosis and this frequently clears in a few weeks.

g. *Renal artery thrombosis.* This is fortunately rare but results in loss of the kidney. It is probably due to a hypercoagulable state from surgery and steroids.

3. *Long-term Complications*

a. *Rejection.* This can occur at any time following transplantation but it is most common in the first 6 months or following any reduction in immunosuppressive therapy. The longer the time from transplantation the less the incidence of acute rejection. It may occur if, however, the patient is unable to take his medications as, for instance, during an episode of vomiting.

Chronic rejection, however, occurs in a number of patients and is due to the deposition of immunoglobulin and inflammatory mediators in the walls of blood vessels and glomeruli. Frequently there is slowly declining renal function accompanied by increasing proteinuria and increasing difficulty in controlling blood pressure. At present there is no effective treatment of chronic rejection.

b. *Recurrent glomerulonephritis.* Some forms of glomerulonephritis such as the dense-deposit variety of mesangiocapillary glomerulonephritis recur in the transplanted kidney. This is frequently impossible to distinguish clinically from chronic rejection and biopsy is needed in such circumstances. As yet there is no satisfactory treatment for recurrent glomerulonephritis.

c. *Infections.* In view of continuing immunosuppressive therapy there is a continued liability to infections. The patient is liable to all forms of bacterial infection and tuberculosis must always be remembered.

The viral infections which give problems are herpes simplex, herpes zoster and cytomegalovirus (CMV). The relationship of CMV infection to rejection is not exactly clear but it appears that if CMV is transferred to the donor in the transplanted kidney there is a considerably increased risk of severe rejection. It would seem prudent therefore not to transplant from CMV-positive donors to CMV-negative recipients.

The fungal infections giving most problems are candida of the upper gastrointestinal tract, aspergillosis of the lung and brain, and cryptococcosis of the central nervous system.

Protozoal infections include toxoplasmosis and *Pneumocystis carinii*. The latter gives rise to progressive pneumonia which used to be termed 'transplant lung'.

d. *Bone disease.* The two major problems are osteoporosis and avascular necrosis. The avascular necrosis occurs in the femoral head and may cause sufficient distress as to warrant hip replacement. It may also occur in the humeral head. The bony problems of uraemia resolve with restoration of satisfactory renal function.

e. *Neoplasia.* This is a problem of prolonged graft survival and long-term immunosuppression. There is an increasing incidence with increasing time from transplant. It occurs mainly in reticulo-endothelial system and skin but other organs such as breast, lung, stomach and liver may be the primary site.

f. *Immunosuppressive drug problems.* In addition to bone disease and neoplasia there are other complications of long-term steroid and azathioprine use. Steroids may give rise to a *proximal myopathy* and/or *cataract*. Fortunately these produce little serious problem for the patient as they rarely progress once the dose is reduced to 15 mg or less daily. Azathioprine may produce a hepatitis by a sensitivity reaction and may rarely be responsible for a pure red cell aplasia. Fortunately both these respond satisfactorily to a change to cyclophosphamide.

g. *Hypertension.* This may continue to be a problem after transplantation or it may appear for the first time. It may be due to excessive renin secretion from the patient's own kidneys or from the transplant consequent on vascular problems. This is best resolved by selective sampling of venous blood for renin assay and investigation of the graft blood supply by isotopes and arteriography.

h. *Local effects.* The transplanted kidney may produce local effects as manifest by the frequency of a hydrocele appearing on the same side as the transplant and the development of mild leg oedema on the transplant side.

i. *Skin.* The skin may be involved in infections:
Bacterial  :  acne
Fungal     :  tinea versicolor

Viral      :   verrucae
           herpes simplex
           herpes zoster

and also in neoplasia:

Keratoacanthoma
Squamous-cell carcinoma
Basal-cell carcinoma

PROGNOSIS. The life expectancy has increased in the past ten years due to experience in controlling rejection, the improved selection of patients and also due to increased expertise from the increased transplantation rate. The prognosis depends upon many factors but current figures would indicate that:

1. In identical twins a greater than 90 per cent graft survival at 5 years.
2. In living related donors an 80 per cent graft survival at 5 years, the results being slightly better for transplants between siblings and slightly worse when from parent to child.
3. In cadaver grafts a 50 per cent graft survival at 5 years.

Patient survival has improved because of the greater willingness to abandon grafts with serious rejection and poor function. The patient is quickly returned to dialysis and rehabilitated in preparation for a potential second transplant. This policy has considerably reduced the number of patients dying from excessive immunosuppressive therapy.

## INTEGRATED APPROACH TO THE MANAGEMENT OF CHRONIC RENAL FAILURE

The management of chronic renal failure has changed considerably in the past twenty years. There are now means of replacing renal function by artificial devices and by transplantation. The various techniques all have advantages and disadvantages and it is important to have a flexible approach to management so that the most appropriate form of therapy is employed. This may mean that the therapy has to be constantly reviewed as a patient's circumstances may change with time.

The first step in the management of a patient with end-stage renal failure is to decide whether replacement therapy is to be offered. As already discussed this will include the majority of patients. The second decision is whether the initial form of therapy should be peritoneal dialysis or haemodialysis. If haemodialysis is favoured then an arteriovenous fistula should be inserted prior to dialysis becoming essential. If peritoneal dialysis is preferred a soft indwelling cannula is inserted at the time dialysis is required.

Once the patient is started on replacement therapy an assessment of the suitability for hospital, satellite or home dialysis should be undertaken.

Also in this rehabilitation phase the suitability for transplantation should be investigated. Thereafter transplantation should be considered for all suitable patients regardless of their mode of replacement therapy. It may be necessary to change patients from one form of treatment to another due to changed circumstances, e.g. a patient on continuous ambulatory peritoneal dialysis (CAPD) may develop complications requiring the transfer to haemodialysis while another patient on haemodialysis may develop such severe vascular access problem that they require transfer to CAPD. In addition, following transplantation, rejection may necessitate a return to dialysis which in the first instance is likely to be hospital based with a subsequent transfer to satellite or home when possible. This flexible approach allows for the best use of all available resources so that the maximum number of patients benefit from the available facilities.

**Integrated Approach, Suggested Scheme**

| | |
|---|---|
| DECISION 1 | Advisability of supportive therapy? |
| DECISION 2 | If answer to 1 is 'yes', then peritoneal or haemodialysis? |
| DECISION 3 | If answer to 2 is for haemodialysis, then hospital, satellite or home based? |
| DECISION 4 | After initial rehabilitation, suitability for transplantation? |
| DECISION 5 | Regular review, is the patient receiving the most appropriate and beneficial form of therapy? |
| | If answer to 5 is 'no', then change. |

# Chapter 9

# GLOMERULONEPHRITIS

Introduction – Diffuse proliferative glomerulonephritis – Mesangiocapillary glomerulonephritis – Membranous glomerulonephritis – Minimal lesion glomerulonephritis – Focal glomerulonephritis – Rapidly progressive (crescentic) glomerulonephritis – Focal glomerulosclerosis

## INTRODUCTION

Glomerulonephritis can be considered as a primary lesion or it may develop secondary to some underlying systemic disease.

**Primary**
>  Diffuse proliferative
>>  Post-streptococcal glomerulonephritis
>>  Mesangial IgG/IgA disease
>  Mesangiocapillary
>>  Subendothelial type
>>  Dense-deposit type
>  Membranous
>  Minimal lesion
>  Focal
>  Rapidly progressive (crescentic)
>>  Goodpasture's syndrome
>  Focal glomerulosclerosis

**Secondary**
>  Systemic lupus erythematosus
>  Polyarteritis
>>  Nodosa type
>>  Microscopic type
>  Wegener's granulomatosis
>  Henoch–Schönlein disease
>  Diabetes mellitus
>  Amyloid

The differentiation into primary and secondary is somewhat artificial but provides a good structure for classification.

The classification of glomerulonephritis depends in most instances on the underlying histological appearances and to understand the pathology a clear understanding of the normal microscopic structure is essential (*see* Chapter 1). In describing the pathological findings the following terms are used:

>  Diffuse: a condition involving all glomeruli.
>  Focal: involvement of some glomeruli while others appear normal.
>  Segmental: involvement of some parts of a glomerular tuft while the remaining part appears normal.

Proliferative: an increase in the number of cells in the glomerular tuft, usually the mesangial cells but also the endothelial cells and the parietal epithelial cells.

Membranous: a thickening of the glomerular capillary wall by sub-endothelial, intramembranous or subepithelial deposits.

Mesangiocapillary: proliferation of cells and thickening of the glomerular capillary wall.

Crescents: proliferation of the epithelial cells of Bowman's capsule. These may be small or large enough to surround the glomerular tuft completely.

The clinical presentation of glomerular disease is variable but the hallmarks are proteinuria, haematuria and hypertension. The following syndromes are recognized modes of presentation:

Acute nephritis
Nephrotic syndrome
Asymptomatic proteinuria
Recurrent haematuria
Hypertension
Acute renal failure
Chronic renal failure

Unfortunately there is no good correlation between clinical findings and underlying pathology. For this reason a definitive diagnosis can only be made by renal biopsy. Most information can be obtained by submitting the biopsy to light microscopy, electron microscopy and immuno-fluorescence.


## DIFFUSE PROLIFERATIVE GLOMERULONEPHRITIS

**Definition.** A diffuse increase in the glomerular cellularity due to a proliferation of mesangial cells frequently associated with an increase in mesangial matrix.

**Presentation.** Extremely variable but typically presents as acute nephritis although a significant number may present as nephrotic syndrome. Patients, particularly mild cases, may also be detected by finding proteinuria at routine examination. In a small number of cases the presentation is with hypertension and/or chronic renal failure.

**Age/Sex Distribution.** May occur at any age and there is no preponderance.

**Clinical Features.** These will depend to a large extent on the severity of the condition. Proteinuria is universal and in the vast majority of cases is unselective. In some patients it may be sufficient to produce nephrotic syndrome. Haematuria is common although it may only be microscopic and intermittent; red blood cell casts may be present and should always be looked for as they will certainly confirm glomerular disease. Hypertension occurs in approximately half the cases and will depend on the severity of the underlying disease. Renal failure is variable and unpredictable and so follow-up of patients is to be recommended.

**Laboratory Findings.** Urinalysis reveals proteinuria in all cases and haematuria in most. Evidence of renal failure depends upon the severity of the case. Plasma proteins may be reduced if the proteinuria exceeds approximately 3 g daily in the adult patient. The typical biochemical findings of low albumin, raised globulins and raised cholesterol will occur in the nephrotic cases. In acute phases of the illness the plasma complement $(C_3)$ may be reduced although in many complement studies will be normal. The ESR is frequently elevated.

**Biopsy Findings.** There is a diffuse proliferation of mesangial cells frequently associated with an increase in mesangial matrix. Occasionally endothelial cells are swollen. There is a wide spectrum of changes from a *mild* or *minor* proliferation of cells with a slight increase in mesangial matrix, a *moderate* proliferation where there is a more marked increase in cells with some endothelial swelling to an *exudative* lesion where there is proliferation associated with the infiltration of polymorphs and the formation of occasional crescents. This is sometimes described as an active or acute nephritis. A progressive lesion is suggested by the finding of areas of hyalinization in glomeruli.

Immunofluorescence frequently shows the presence of immunoglobulins, complement components and fibrin in glomeruli. Electron microscopy demonstrates deposition of material in glomerular capillary walls and the mesangium. In cases where there are circulating soluble immune complexes there may be found subepithelial deposits of electron dense material – 'humps' – thought to be aggregations of antigen–antibody complexes.

**Diagnosis.** This can be suspected on the clinical features, particularly if there has been a documented preceding streptococcal infection, but can only be confirmed by biopsy and the exclusion of systemic diseases which may produce proliferative glomerulonephritis.

**Aetiology.** The majority of cases are thought to be due to the deposition of small soluble circulating immune complexes in glomerular capillary walls. Classically this disease is typified by the occurrence of a streptococcal infection, usually of the throat or skin, followed some 10–14 days later by the development of acute nephritis. However, the number of cases which can be attributed to the streptococcal antigen is disappointingly small and it is highly likely that there are many antigens which can initiate this reaction. Searches for circulating immune complexes have also been disappointing but this may reflect the inadequacy of our methods for detection rather than the lack of complexes.

**Pathogenesis.** Antigens will stimulate the production of antibodies and providing the type of antibody is right and there are approximately equal amounts of antigen and antibody there will be the formation of small soluble complexes. These are deposited in the glomerular capillary walls and result in the activation of the complement cascade. The consequence of this is the attraction of polymorphs with the liberation of kinins and other enzymes which stimulate endothelial swelling, platelet aggregation and fibrin formation. This inflammatory response produces the glomerulo-nephritis. Providing the antigen is eliminated and the formation of complexes ceases then there is a high probability that the inflammatory lesion will resolve and the glomeruli return to normality. However, if the deposition of complexes continues or the glomerulus is unable to cope with the inflammatory material then a progressive lesion is likely to develop. Crescent formation is considered to be a reaction to the extrusion of blood from the glomerular capillary into the urinary space and therefore may indicate the severity of the capillary wall lesion.

**Natural History.** This is extremely variable and to a large extent depends upon the degree of glomerular proliferation, the extent of renal functional impairment and the presence of hypertension. The majority of cases make a satisfactory recovery although there may be persistent proteinuria with or without microscopic haematuria. Patients presenting with acute nephritis may either resolve completely, improve but have continuing minor urinary abnormalities, die in the acute stage from renal failure or hypertension, or progress to chronic renal failure. Patients who present with asymptomatic proteinuria usually have a good prognosis but if the presentation is as nephrotic syndrome the outlook is not as good.

Poor prognostic indicators are continuing hypertension, the development of renal functional impairment, circumferential crescents, and the presence of areas of segmental hyalinization in glomeruli.

**Management.** There is no specific therapy. Management should be aimed at:
1. Establishing diagnosis and fully assessing renal function.
2. Controlling hypertension, if present.
3. Giving diuretics if oedema present.
4. Searching for focus of infection and if present treating with appropriate antibiotics.
5. A careful follow-up.


## POST-STREPTOCOCCAL GLOMERULONEPHRITIS

**Definition.** This is a glomerulonephritis which develops consequent on the formation of immune complexes as a result of a streptococcal infection.

**Presentation.** Acute nephritis, a number of patients present as asymptomatic proteinuria and/or haematuria.

**Age/Sex Distribution.** Most common in children of school age but can occur at any age.

**Clinical Features.** Streptococcal infection of skin or throat followed some 10–14 days later by the development of oliguria, smokey urine due to haematuria, hypertension and deterioration in renal function. All four criteria need not be present as hypertension and renal failure is variable. Encephalopathy may occur due to the hypertension, fluid retention or the simultaneous deposition of complexes in the arachnoid of the brain.

**Laboratory Findings.** Proteinuria is usually unselective; haematuria as red blood cell casts; urea and creatinine variably elevated; complement ($C_3$) depressed in acute phase; ASO titre elevated. It may be possible to isolate the streptococcus from the throat, nose or skin but in many instances the original infection will have cleared.

**Biopsy Findings.** The most common finding is of a diffuse exudative proliferative glomerulonephritis although in a small number of patients the biopsy may show a rapidly progressive (crescentic) appearance. On electron microscopy in the acute phase there may be the presence of electron dense subepithelial deposits – 'humps'.

**Pathogenesis.** Following the localization of small soluble complexes containing streptococcal antigen and antibody in the glomerular capillary wall there is activation of the complement cascade with subsequent polymorph attraction, endothelial damage, platelet aggregation and fibrin formation.

**Prognosis.** In 80–90 per cent of children there is a full recovery while in a small number there are continuing urinary abnormalities for many years. In a very small number of patients there may be death from hypertension or renal failure in the acute stage. A small number may progress to renal failure at a later date. There are currently some very long-term follow-up studies of epidemic outbreaks but the results are not yet available. The prognosis is less satisfactory in adults with permanent renal impairment being more common.

**Management**
1. Treat underlying infections.
2. Control hypertension.
3. Monitor renal function and treat appropriately.
4. There does not appear to be any value in long-term antibiotics.
5. Long-term follow-up.


## MESANGIAL IgG/IgA (BERGER'S) DISEASE

**Definition.** A proliferative glomerulonephritis characterized by the deposition of IgG and IgA in the mesangium.

**Presentation.** Recurrent haematuria is the most common mode of presentation although the syndrome is also frequently detected as asymptomatic microscopic haematuria where widespread and routine urinalysis is performed.

**Age/Sex Distribution.** Most commonly occurs in the 15–25-year-old patient. Male preponderance.

**Clinical Features.** There are no marked clinical features. Patients are frequently asymptomatic although their macroscopic haematuria usually occurs in immediate association with some intercurrent infection. Hypertension and renal failure are uncommon.

**Laboratory Investigations.** Renal function is usually normal, proteinuria is variable but seldom greater than 3 g daily. Microscopic haematuria is common.

**Biopsy Findings.** The findings are variable but include, on light microscopy, a mild mesangial proliferation with some increase in mesangial matrix, or a focal and segmental proliferative glomerulonephritis. On immuno-fluorescence microscopy there is mesangial deposition of IgG and IgA with a striking lack of material in capillary walls.

**Diagnosis.** Can only be made with immunofluorescence microscopy.

**Aetiology and Pathogenesis.** Unknown.

**Natural History.** Initial presentation is usually between 15 and 20 years. Many progress with recurrent haematuria for up to 10 years and then resolve. Some 5 per cent progress to renal failure requiring dialysis and/or transplantation.

**Management.** There is no specific treatment. Follow-up is required as there is no way of predicting those who will progress to renal failure.


## MESANGIOCAPILLARY GLOMERULONEPHRITIS

**Definition.** A glomerulonephritis characterized by the proliferation of mesangial cells and the expansion of the mesangial matrix so that the capillary lumina are reduced to peripheral slits and the glomerulus develops a lobular appearance.

**Presentation.** Frequently as acute nephritis although may also present as asymptomatic proteinuria, recurrent haematuria or hypertension. Some cases who present with acute nephritis or asymptomatic proteinuria may proceed to nephrotic syndrome. Rarely patients present with chronic renal failure.

**Age/Sex Distribution.** Most common in the age group 15–25. There is a female preponderance.

**Clinical Features.** There are no specific clinical features.

**Laboratory Findings.** Proteinuria common and unselective. Haematuria common. Raised urea and creatinine common and these increase with time. In approximately 50 per cent of cases there is a persistent hypocomplementaemia. The plasma $C_3$ concentration is low while the $C_4$ concentration is normal indicating alternate pathology activation due to the presence of the nephritic factor. This is thought to be an immunoglobulin. The complement abnormality occurs in the 'dense-deposit' type of mesangiocapillary glomerulonephritis (*vide infra*).

**Biopsy Findings.** On biopsy two types can be identified, 'dense-deposit' and 'subendothelial'. In the subendothelial type there is mesangial cellular proliferation, an increase in mesangial matrix and an interposition of mesangial matrix between the endothelial cells and the glomerular capillary basement membrane. This gives the appearance of splitting of the basement membrane which on light microscopy gives the capillary wall a double contour. In the dense-deposit type there is mesangial cellular proliferation, accumulation of mesangial matrix and, in addition, an irregular thickening of the capillary basement membrane due to the deposition of electron dense material. In both types small crescents may be visible.

**Diagnosis.** By biopsy although persistent hypocomplementaemia ($C_3$) in the presence of a normal $C_4$ is highly suggestive of the dense-deposit type.

**Aetiology and Pathogenesis.** Unknown although in some cases it appears to develop following a bacterial infection.

**Natural History.** The dense-deposit and subendothelial types appear similar clinically. The majority of cases progress to end-stage renal failure over a time span of about five years. Some patients, however, appear to remain in stable renal function for many years. The development of hypertension is a poor prognostic factor. The dense-deposit type may recur in a transplanted kidney.

**Management.** There is no specific treatment.
1. Establish diagnosis.
2. Obtain base-line renal function studies.
3. Control hypertension.
4. Follow-up carefully.
5. Counsel against pregnancy as it is frequently attended by deterioration in renal function. Oral contraceptives should be used with caution.

**Association.** Mesangiocapillary glomerulonephritis of the dense-deposit type frequently occurs in patients with partial lipodystrophy. This is a condition characterized by the symmetrical loss of subcutaneous fat from the upper half of the body while in the lower half there may be a normal or increased amount. It usually develops within a year following a febrile illness in childhood. It is also associated with diabetes mellitus, hepatomegaly and retinitis pigmentosa. The majority of patients (90 per cent) are females and there is a hazard of deterioration of renal function during pregnancy.

## MEMBRANOUS GLOMERULONEPHRITIS

**Definition.** Diffuse uniform thickening of the glomerular capillary wall in all glomeruli.

**Presentation.** Usually as nephrotic syndrome but may be detected as asymptomatic proteinuria.

**Age/Sex Distribution.** Most common in middle age (35–55) and there is a male preponderance (M : F, 3 : 1).

**Clinical Findings.** Gross haematuria is rare but microscopic haematuria common. Hypertension is present in approximately 30 per cent of cases at presentation. Renal failure occurs late.

**Laboratory Findings.** Low plasma albumin with associated increase in globulins and cholesterol. In early stages serum creatinine and blood urea usually normal. Complement studies normal. Proteinuria usually heavy and unselective.

**Biopsy Findings.** This depends to a large extent on the time at which the biopsy is performed. In the early stages there is a diffuse thickening of all glomerular capillary walls with little or no evidence of mesangial cell proliferation. On electron microscopy there is subepithelial deposition of electron-dense material but with time these deposits appear to become incorporated into the basement membrane, frequently becoming electron-lucent. Immunofluorescence shows the presence of immunoglobulins and complement in the deposits but in late stages of the disease no immunofluorescence may be detected.

**Diagnosis.** A membranous glomerulonephritis may be associated with a number of conditions (*vide infra*) but in the majority of cases is idiopathic. The diagnosis, therefore, can only be made on biopsy findings.

**Pathogenesis.** The deposition of electron-dense deposits in a subepithelial position is highly suggestive of an immune-complex mediated disease. This is supported by the fact that a number of cases are associated with conditions where it is possible that antigens are repeatedly released into the circulation, e.g. malaria, syphilis, malignant disease.

**Natural History.** If the membranous lesion develops in association with a bacterial, viral or protozoal infection then the prognosis is to a large extent dependent upon the underlying infection. In idiopathic cases some 60 per cent show a slow, steady decline in renal function with progression to renal failure. (Approximately 50 per cent die from renal failure within 10 years of diagnosis.) A number of patients (approximately 10 per cent) recover completely while the remainder continue with persistent proteinuria but stable renal function.

**Management**
1. High protein, low sodium diet providing renal function is not seriously impaired.
2. Diuretic therapy.
3. Regular follow-up to detect any change in renal function.
4. Various treatment schedules including prednisone, azathioprine, chlorambucil or cyclophosphamide have been suggested but at present there is no clear evidence that these are of value.

**Clinical Associations.** May be found in:
1. Idiopathic cases, where no underlying aetiology can be identified.
2. Infections, malaria, persistent hepatitis B antigenaemia, syphilis.
3. Drug complications, penicillamine, gold, heavy metals.
4. Neoplasia, particularly carcinomas of stomach and breast, Hodgkin's disease.
5. Sarcoidosis, diabetes mellitus.

**Renal Vein Thrombosis and Membranous Glomerulonephritis.** It has been suggested that renal vein thrombosis will produce a membranous glomerular lesion. It is now considered that the renal vein thrombosis is due to a hypercoagulable state which frequently develops in nephrotic patients and thus the thrombosis is a result of the membranous glomerulonephritis and not a cause.


## MINIMAL LESION GLOMERULONEPHRITIS

**Definition.** This is a syndrome characterized by severe proteinuria, and the presence of only minimal abnormalities on renal biopsy.

**Presentation.** Most commonly as nephrotic syndrome but on rare occasions is detected as asymptomatic proteinuria. There may be a history of previous upper respiratory tract infection, atopic allergy, recent exposure to extrinsic allergens or immunization.

**Age/Sex Distribution.** Affects children (aged 3–12) predominantly with a slight male preponderance. It does, however, affect adults.

**Clinical Findings.** Haematuria and hypertension are both rare. Renal failure is uncommon but may occur in severe cases when there is marked hypovolaemia. Patients frequently have atopic conditions.

**Laboratory Findings.** Low plasma albumin with associated increase in $\beta_2$-globulins and cholesterol. Serum creatinine and blood urea usually normal. Proteinuria is usually heavy and selective. Complement studies normal.

**Biopsy Findings.** On light microscopy the glomeruli appear normal but may show a slight degree of proliferation of mesangial cells and increase is mesangial matrix. Tubular cells may show lipid droplets (lipid nephrosis) and foam cells may be present in the interstitium. Immunofluorescence microscopy is usually negative but may demonstrate very small amounts of IgM and occasionally $C_3$. On electron microscopy there is a characteristic loss of epithelial cell foot processes and a 'smearing' of the cell along the capillary basement membrane.

**Diagnosis.** Depends upon:
1. The exclusion of other glomerular disease.
2. The presence of selective proteinuria.
3. Typical biopsy findings.
4. Steroid responsiveness.

**Pathogenesis.** Presently unknown but there are suggestions of an altered T-cell function.

**Natural History.** Normally follows a remitting and relapsing course. Spontaneous remission occurs in approximately 30 per cent of children and 10 per cent of adults.

**Management**
1. Diuretics to reduce oedema.
2. Biopsy to determine correct diagnosis.
3. Steroid therapy, 1 mg/kg/day or 2 mg/kg/alternate day. If the urine is free from protein for 2 weeks, or 2 months elapse without response, prednisone should be gradually reduced. When relapses are frequent or unacceptable steroid toxicity develops then cyclophosphamide (2 mg/kg) should be used.
4. Regular follow-up to detect relapses at an early stage.

**Complications.** In the untreated patient complications include increased incidence of infection (particularly skin) and thromboembolism.


## FOCAL GLOMERULONEPHRITIS

**Definition.** A condition characterized by glomerular changes in some glomeruli while others appear normal. It is found frequently in systemic diseases but also occurs in the absence of any systemic disease.

**Presentation.** Most frequently as recurrent haematuria but may also present as acute nephritis or nephrotic syndrome.

**Age/Sex Distribution.** Occurs mainly in young adults, 15–30 years old. Slight male preponderance.

**Clinical Features.** In patients with systemic disease the clinical features will depend entirely on the underlying disease. In others macroscopic haematuria frequently immediately follows some febrile illness while between episodes microscopic haematuria is present. Proteinuria is usually mild and hypertension or renal impairment is rare.

**Laboratory Findings.** Usually no abnormality detected.

**Biopsy Findings.** On light microscopy some glomeruli appear affected while the remainder are normal. The percentage of glomeruli affected is variable. In glomeruli the changes, usually proliferative, are frequently confined to one or two lobules and usually found at the periphery of the lobule. Small crescents are occasionally found. In some cases, particularly those associated with microscopic polyarteritis, the glomerular changes may show areas of necrosis.

**Aetiology and Pathogenesis.** Unknown.

**Natural History.** The prognosis is usually good. In many instances the episodes of recurrent haematuria will resolve and renal function is unaffected. In a small number of patients progressive renal impairment occurs. In those associated with systemic diseases the prognosis will depend entirely on the underlying disease.

**Management.** There is no specific therapy.
1. Establish diagnosis.
2. Assess renal function.
3. Exclude systemic disease.
4. Careful follow-up to detect the small number which may progress to renal failure.

**Associations.** A focal proliferative or necrotizing glomerulonephritis may be found in a considerable number of conditions and these should be confirmed by appropriate investigations. Usually evidence of systemic disease precedes the appearance of renal involvement but this is not invariable. Focal glomerular lesions are recognized in the following:
Systemic lupus erythematosus
Microscopic polyarteritis
Henoch–Schönlein syndrome
Bacterial endocarditis
Mesangial IgG/IgA disease
Goodpasture's syndrome
Heroin nephropathy.


## RAPIDLY PROGRESSIVE (CRESCENTIC) GLOMERULONEPHRITIS

**Definition.** A glomerulonephritis usually presenting as an acute reduction in renal function, progressing rapidly to uraemia and characterized by large circumferential crescents in 70 per cent or more of glomeruli.

**Presentation.** Most commonly as acute renal failure without obvious cause.

**Age/Sex Distribution.** Can occur at any age but is most common in older adults.

**Clinical Features.** Are mainly those of acute renal failure such as oliguria, pulmonary oedema or cardiac failure. Hypertension is variable. Some have a non-specific illness and are found to be uraemic during investigation.

**Laboratory Findings.** Raised urea and creatinine associated with a metabolic acidosis. Haematuria and proteinuria common. Complement usually normal. Plasma proteins normal.

**Biopsy Findings.** There may be little or no proliferation of the glomerular tuft but there is parietal epithelial cell proliferation producing large circumferential crescents in 70 per cent or more glomeruli. The tubules are frequently ischaemic and the interstitium is oedematous and contains inflammatory cells.

**Diagnosis.** From renal biopsy and exclusion of other conditions (*vide infra*).

**Aetiology.** May rarely follow a streptococcal or viral infection but in the vast majority of patients no cause can be found.

**Pathogenesis.** As for proliferative glomerulonephritis.

**Prognosis.** Extremely poor.

**Management**
1. As for acute renal failure (*see* Chapter 7).
2. In view of poor prognosis 1 g of methylprednisolone (Solu-medrone) i.v. daily for 3 days followed by high dose steroids.
3. If renal function deteriorating then plasmapheresis may halt the decline but its use is still experimental.

**Clinical Associations.** A crescentic glomerulonephritis may be found in:
Goodpasture's syndrome (*see below*)
Systemic lupus erythematosus (p. 112)
Wegener's granulomatosis (p. 118)
Microscopic polyarteritis (p. 116)
Henoch--Schönlein syndrome (p. 121)
and so investigations must be undertaken to detect these conditions.


## GOODPASTURE'S SYNDROME

**Definition.** This is a variant of rapidly progressive glomerulonephritis where there is the presence of circulating antiglomerular basement membrane (GBM) antibody.

**Presentation.** Usually as acute renal failure but it may be detected during investigation of anaemia or haemoptysis.

**Age/Sex Distribution.** Affects mainly young adult males.

**Clinical Findings.** There may be a history of recent viral or bacterial respiratory infection or exposure to hydrocarbons. Gross haematuria may be the first sign. Haemoptysis is frequently but not invariably present. Renal symptoms usually occur first but in some patients the lungs appear to be involved first.

**Laboratory Findings.** The findings are frequently those of acute renal failure, oliguria, rising urea and creatinine. The diagnostic finding is the detection of anti-GBM antibody in the serum.

**Biopsy Findings.** In early stages there may be a focal necrotizing glomerular lesion while in later stages the appearance is that of a rapidly progressive (crescentic) glomerulonephritis. Immunofluorescence microscopy reveals a linear deposition of IgG and frequent $C_3$ in glomerular capillary walls. A similar linear deposition may be found on alveolar basement membranes.

**Diagnosis.** This is made by the detection of anti-GBM antibody and the clinical findings.

**Pathogenesis.** The renal and pulmonary lesions are due to the effect of the anti-GBM antibody. The lung tissue appears to share common antigens with glomerular basement membrane.

**Natural History.** Untreated, progresses rapidly to death either from renal failure or pulmonary haemorrhage.

### Management
1. Diagnosis must be established as soon as possible.
2. Acute renal failure treated along conventional lines (*see* Chapter 7).
3. Plasmapheresis combined with immunosuppression (prednisone, azathioprine and cyclophosphamide).
4. High-dose steroids may be required to control pulmonary haemorrhage.
5. If renal function is destroyed then long-term dialysis and possible transplantation. It is important to know that there is no anti-GBM antibody present at the time of transplantation.


## FOCAL GLOMERULOSCLEROSIS

**Definition.** This is a syndrome which commonly has a nephrotic presentation and in which renal biopsy shows focal areas of sclerosis in glomeruli.

**Presentation.** Most commonly as nephrotic syndrome and in early cases is indistinguishable from minimal lesion glomerulonephritis.

**Age/Sex Distribution.** Occurs at all ages but there is a peak incidence of onset in the third decade.

**Clinical Findings.** Haematuria is rare. Hypertension, if present, occurs at a late stage. Renal failure is uncommon at presentation but develops as time progresses.

**Laboratory Findings.** Low plasma albumin with associated increase in $\beta_2$-globulins and cholesterol. Creatinine and urea may be elevated in late cases. Complement studies normal. Proteinuria usually heavy and unselective.

**Biopsy Findings.** This depends upon the stage of the illness at which biopsy is performed. Initially only the juxtamedullary glomeruli are involved but with time the lesions become apparent in those more peripheral. In glomeruli there are segmental areas of sclerosis without proliferation or necrosis. The sclerotic areas gradually expand and obliterate all capillaries in the glomeruli. Focal tubular atrophy with some interstitial inflammation occurs. Immunofluorescence microscopy often shows deposition of IgM and $C_3$ in affected glomeruli. Electron microscopy shows enlargement of mesangial regions containing dense deposits in sclerotic lobules.

**Diagnosis.** Can only be made on the biopsy findings.

**Pathogenesis.** Unknown.

**Natural History.** The nephrotic presentation may run a relapsing and remitting course. In more than 50 per cent of patients there is a steady decline in renal function progressing to renal failure. The lesion may reappear in a transplanted kidney.

**Management**
1.  High protein, low sodium diet.
2.  Diuretics to reduce oedema.
3.  Regular follow-up to detect declining renal function and take appropriate action.
4.  There is at present no convincing evidence that steroids or immuno-suppressive agents are of any value.

**Clinical Associations.** May be found in association with heroin addiction.

# Chapter 10

# THE KIDNEY IN SYSTEMIC DISEASE

General introduction – Systemic lupus erythematosus – Polyarteritis – Wegener's granulomatosis – Rheumatoid arthritis – Scleroderma (systemic sclerosis) – Amyloidosis – Henoch–Schönlein syndrome (anaphylactoid purpura) – Diabetes mellitus – Gout – Sarcoidosis – Subacute bacterial endocarditis

## GENERAL INTRODUCTION

In many patients with glomerulonephritis it is the glomerular disease which appears to be the primary problem, with the associated hypertension and renal failure as secondary phenomena. There is, however, a group of conditions in which the glomerular lesion is only one feature of a more widespread disease process. In such cases the glomerulonephritis can be considered *secondary* although it must be remembered that in many cases the renal involvement is of considerable importance and may be the ultimate cause of death.

The majority of conditions fall into the so-called 'connective tissue diseases' group, e.g. systemic lupus erythematosus, polyarteritis and scleroderma, while others are of a metabolic nature, e.g. amyloidosis and diabetes mellitus.

## SYSTEMIC LUPUS ERYTHEMATOSUS

Systemic lupus erythematosus (SLE) is a multisystem disease which may present in many ways and affect every system in the body. It is frequently difficult to differentiate from other connective tissue disorders and its clinical presentations are numerous. Renal involvement occurs in approximately 75 per cent of SLE patients and carries a poor prognosis. It frequently appears early in the natural history but it must be remembered that it can occur at any time.

**Aetiology.** In spite of much research the aetiology of SLE remains uncertain. The possible causes are:
1. A viral infection; there has, however, been no satisfactory isolation of a specific virus although virus-like particles have been visualized on electron microscopy.
2. An autoimmune state exists but this does not explain how or why the disease starts.
3. An inherited immunological deficiency; this is supported by the familial incidence and the increased incidence of HLA-8.

**Pathogenesis.** The development of renal disease is due to the deposition of antigen–antibody complexes in the glomerulus. This is associated with complement activation, endothelial damage and subsequent fibrinogen activation with the formation of fibrin and thrombi.

**Pathology**

GLOMERULAR CHANGES. The glomerular changes can be divided into several recognizable forms.

1. Minor changes (30 per cent). In a number of patients the glomeruli appear relatively normal on light microscopy. There may be minor increase in mesangial cells in some segments with or without focal thickening of the capillary wall.

2. Focal glomerulonephritis (20 per cent). There is segmental proliferation of cells which in some glomeruli may even show focal necrosis. Remaining segments of glomeruli and other glomeruli may appear normal.

3. Diffuse proliferative glomerulonephritis (35 per cent). This may vary in severity from a mild proliferation of mesangial cells to necrosis and crescent formation. On electron microscopy subendothelial deposits are seen and on immunofluorescence these are frequently shown to contain IgG, complement and fibrin.

4. Membranous glomerulonephritis (15 per cent). There is diffuse generalized thickening of the capillary wall essentially indistinguishable from idiopathic membranous glomerulonephritis. Electron microscopy reveals subendothelial deposits which can be demonstrated to contain IgG and complement.

5. Haematoxylin bodies are specific to SLE and are probably the disordered nuclei of cells damaged by auto-antibodies.

6. Wire-loop lesions in capillary walls are highly suggestive of SLE although they may occur rarely in other conditions.

VASCULAR CHANGES. Thickening of arteriolar walls and fibrinoid necrosis are frequently observed.

INTERSTITIAL CHANGES. Patchy fibrosis is seen particularly in longstanding cases and probably represents the effect of glomerular loss and/or vascular occlusions.

**Clinical Features.** A characteristic feature of SLE is its multisystem involvement. It may therefore present in many ways. The renal manifestations are:

1. Proteinuria – the most common sign. It may be asymptomatic or sufficient to produce the nephrotic syndrome. It is usually greatest in cases with a diffuse proliferative or a membranous appearance on microscopy.

2. Haematuria is common and usually microscopic.

3. Hypertension occurs in approximately 20 per cent of patients with SLE but this incidence is greater in those with renal involvement.

4. Renal failure may present as an acute or chronic illness.

5. Renal involvement may not be manifest when a diagnosis of SLE is

established but it may develop at any time during the course of the disease.
6.  SLE is a disease of remission and exacerbation and thus the clinical features are liable to change.

**Diagnostic Criteria.** The diagnosis of lupus erythematosus can be difficult due to the considerable overlap of the various 'connective-tissue' syndromes. The American Rheumatism Association listed fourteen manifestations of SLE and suggested that a diagnosis could be made if four or more were present. The manifestations are:
1.  Facial erythema (butterfly rash).
2.  Discoid lupus.
3.  Raynaud's phenomenon.
4.  Alopecia.
5.  Photosensitivity.
6.  Oral or nasopharyngeal ulceration.
7.  Arthritis without deformity.
8.  Lupus erythematosus cells.
9.  Chronic false positive serological test for syphilis.
10.  Profuse proteinuria.
11.  Cellular casts on urine microscopy.
12.  Pleurisy and/or pericarditis.
13.  Psychosis and/or convulsions.
14.  Haemolytic anaemia and/or leucopenia and/or thrombocytopenia.

Since the publication of this list in 1971 improvements in serological tests have been made and many would now consider a diagnosis established on the finding of a high titre of anti-DNA antibodies particularly when associated with low plasma $C_3$ concentration and a compatible renal biopsy.

**Indications for Renal Biopsy**
1.  To confirm or establish a diagnosis in patients considered to have SLE.
2.  To determine the histological type as a guide to prognosis (*vide infra*).
3.  To determine the effects of therapy.

**Management.** The management of any disease which has remissions and exacerbations is likely to prove difficult. In spite of this considerable improvement in prognosis has been made in recent years.
1.  Establish diagnosis.
2.  Establish baseline studies; renal function, proteinuria, haemoglobin, WBC, platelet count, ESR, complement ($C_3$) and DNA binding.
3.  Obtain renal biopsy to determine histological type.
4.  Drug treatment depends upon the severity and clinical manifestations. In mild disease and where there is no renal involvement

salicylates, indomethacin and phenylbutazone are of value. Anti-malarials are of value, particularly for skin manifestations.

5. Steroids must be used for patients with renal disease and for severe manifestations such as haemolytic anaemia, thrombocytopenic purpura, central nervous system involvement, acute vasculitis and severe arthropathy.

   Steroid therapy should be commenced in a dose of 40–80 mg daily and maintained for two months. The dose can then be slowly reduced (a useful guide is approximately 10 per cent every 10 days) until a maintenance dose is determined. During this time a careful watch needs to be kept on the clinical status, the ESR and plasma $C_3$. In patients requiring less then 20 mg daily of prednisone the addition of an antimalarial may allow for a reduction in steroid dose. In patients requiring more than 20 mg daily of prednisone consideration should be given to an alternate-day regime. In view of the high incidence of side effects, treatment can be started with an alternate-day regimen or patients can be converted at a later stage in their course. In alternate-day therapy the requirement is for approximately 20 per cent greater than twice the daily dose (i.e. a patient requiring 20 mg daily of prednisone will probably need 50 mg in alternate days).

   In very severe cases it may be of value to commence therapy with intravenous high-dose steroids such as 1 g methylprednisolone (Solu-medrone) daily for 3 days.

6. Frequent and detailed follow-up is required.
7. Immunosuppressive drugs such as azathioprine and cyclophospha-mide have been used but as yet there is no clear indication of their value.
8. Plasmapheresis has been used to remove the antibody and/or com-plexes and may be of value in cases where high dose steroids seem to be inadequate.
9. In patients with renal involvement hypertension may develop and in such patients although both methyldopa (Aldomet) and hydral-azine (Apresoline) have been implicated in producing SLE they may be used.
10. If end-stage renal failure occurs dialysis and subsequent trans-plantation should be considered. There is, however, a higher incidence of hypertension and infection in these patients.

**Prognosis.** The prognosis is variable and to a large extent depends upon the type and severity of the renal involvement.

1. In those patients with normal histology or minor changes the prognosis is very good although it must be remembered that renal involvement may develop at any time.
2. Focal glomerulonephritis indicates a relatively benign course and the

5-year survival is approximately 65 per cent. The requirement for steroids is usually low. Most patients die from non-renal causes. The change to a diffuse histological picture can occur but only rarely.

3. Diffuse proliferative appearances have a poor prognosis with approximately a 25 per cent 5-year survival. Most patients die from renal involvement. The requirement for steroid is high. The severity of the glomerular appearance, particularly the amount of subendothelial deposits, correlates well with the prognosis.

4. Membranous forms of SLE have a good prognosis. The 5-year survival is approximately 85 per cent. The requirement for steroids is low. A presentation of nephrotic syndrome is a poor prognostic indicator. Renal failure, if it arises, usually develops slowly. Death is usually due to non-renal causes.

5. Patients who at the time of presentation, regardless of histology, have severe hypertension or a creatine clearance of less than 20 ml/l have a poor prognosis.

**Drug-induced Systemic Lupus Erythematosus.** A wide variety of drugs have been reported as causing SLE but the most common are:

Hydralazine
Procainamide
Methyldopa
Chlorpromazine

The incidence of renal involvement in drug-induced SLE is low and in the majority of patients the clinical and laboratory manifestations regress after cessation of the drug involved.


## POLYARTERITIS

**Introduction.** Two types of polyarteritis are recognized, polyarteritis nodosa (classic polyarteritis) where medium-sized muscular arteries are involved, and microscopic polyarteritis where capillaries and in particular glomerular capillaries are involved. In both forms renal involvement is common and of serious prognosis.

**Aetiology.** It is most likely that this condition is a manifestation of a hypersensitivity reaction. Experimentally produced serum sickness causes pathological changes similar to polyarteritis.

Certain drugs – sulphonamides, thiouracil and penicillin – have been reported as causing a hypersensitivity reaction with subsequent polyarteritis. Some reports indicate that hepatitis B antigen (Australia antigen) can cause this syndrome but the evidence is as yet unconvincing.

**Pathogenesis.** The pathogenesis is not clear. It is most likely due to the action of immune complexes and the two forms of the syndrome may represent the production of complexes of different sizes. However, in some patients no immunoglobulins can be found in the lesions and therefore other pathogenetic mechanisms may operate.

**Pathology**

    A. NODOSA FORM. Large, muscular arteries are involved and the appearances will, to a large extent, depend on the stage of the development of the lesion. The most prominent features in the acute stage are fibrinoid necrosis and perivascular accumulation of polymorphs, mononuclear cells and eosinophils. In severe cases infarction of tissue distal to the vascular lesion occurs. Thrombosis of affected vessels may occur.

    B. MICROSCOPIC FORM. In the kidney the most prominent lesion is in the glomeruli. The appearances may be variable and in mild cases are focal and segmental. Fibrinoid necrosis may affect a few capillary loops or a lobule. There is frequently cellular proliferation and crescents are common. Appearances identical to rapidly progressive glomerulonephritis (Chapter 9) may be found.

    Tubular changes are not marked except in severe forms and blood vessels are relatively spared.

**Clinical Features.** The clinical features to some extent depend on the type of polyarteritis but both are:
1. More common in males (male : female, 2 : 1).
2. More common in middle-aged and older patients.
3. Associated with fever, arthropathy and generalized malaise.
4. Associated with anaemia, high ESR and eosinophilia.

A. NODOSA FORM
1. Hypertension is a common finding and may rapidly progress to a malignant phase.
2. Loin pain may occur due to areas of renal infarction.
3. Macroscopic haematuria.

B. MICROSCOPIC FORM
1. Hypertension is much less common.
2. Clinical presentation is usually as either acute nephritis or in severe cases, acute renal failure.
3. Haematuria is usually microscopic.

**Diagnosis.** The diagnosis can only be made with any certainty on histological grounds. In the nodosa form renal arteriography may be of considerable value in demonstrating multiple small aneurysms in the muscular arteries and/or associated areas of ischaemia or infarction. Biopsy in the nodosa form may not reveal any vascular changes due to the patchy nature of the lesion.

A diagnosis of the microscopic form is more difficult and is made by the combination of a typical clinical history, multisystem involvement, high ESR, eosinophilia and a compatible glomerular lesion.

**Management**
1. Establish diagnosis as soon as possible. In patients with severe renal involvement treatment is a matter of urgency.
2. Obtain baseline studies of renal function and haematology.
3. Steroids are essential. The dose will depend upon the severity, but is usually between 60–100 mg daily of prednisone. In cases with severe glomerular changes it may be of value to start treatment with methylprednisolone (Solu-medrone) 1 g daily i.v. for 3 days. High-dose steroids should be maintained for 2 months and then gradually reduced. Maintenance therapy will vary between 10 and 30 mg daily of prednisone, If more than 20 mg daily are required an alternate-day regimen should be considered in an attempt to reduce steroid toxicity.
4. Frequent follow-up to monitor progress is mandatory.
5. Hypertension and renal failure should be treated as and when required.

**Prognosis.** Renal failure is the commonest cause of death in patients with polyarteritis.

Steroid therapy is of undoubted value but a number of patients appear to relapse after several years in spite of apparently successful therapy. The more severe the renal involvement the poorer the prognosis.


## WEGENER'S GRANULOMATOSIS

This is probably a variant of polyarteritis and is characterized by:
1. Granulomatous lesions in the upper respiratory tract and lungs.
2. Fibrinoid necrosis of blood vessels.
3. Focal proliferative glomerulonecrosis.

The clinical presentation is usually initially due to nasal symptoms, chronic cough, haemoptysis or pleurisy. Renal manifestations occur later and in many cases the renal involvement is only detected during the course of investigation of the respiratory symptoms. Renal failure is common.

Diagnosis is made by a combination of chest X-ray, biopsy of lesion in the respiratory tract and renal biopsy.

The management and prognosis have altered considerably. Prolonged remission can be produced by therapy with either cyclophosphamide or azathioprine with or without the addition of steroids.

The aetiology is unknown.


## RHEUMATOID ARTHRITIS

Renal involvement in rheumatoid arthritis is more common than one would suspect. The lesions which may arise in such patients are:
1. *Amyloidosis:* This probably occurs to some extent in the kidney of

approximately 20 per cent of patients. The reason for this high incidence is not known, but may be related to the immunoglobulin abnormalities and also the increased incidence of infection.

2. *Mild Proliferative Glomerulonephritis:* This has been reported in several series but the importance is unknown.
3. *Arteritis:* Lesion similar to those found in other organs may be present.
4. *Interstitial Nephritis:* This is most likely associated with analgesic therapy and in severe cases may produce *papillary necrosis.*
5. *Complications of Therapy: Gold* has been widely used in rheumatoid arthritis and it may produce either a proximal tubular cellular damage or a lesion rather like membranous glomerulonephritis although the membrane involvement may be patchy. *Penicillamine* has also been used widely and this produces a membranous nephropathy in approximately 20 per cent of cases.

## SCLERODERMA (SYSTEMIC SCLEROSIS)

This is an unusual condition of unknown aetiology in which there is widespread vascular disease, which is more common in females than males, which tends to occur in middle age and which frequently affects the kidney.

**Clinical Features.** The initial manifestations are usually in the skin and gastrointestinal tract. Raynaud's phenomenon and a thickening and tightening of the skin, particularly in the fingers and around the mouth, are common. Dysphagia may occur.

Renal manifestations may occur early as a mild proteinuria but more frequently present as a terminal event by acute renal failure. Hypertension, even to the point of malignant hypertension, may precede the acute episode.

**Pathology.** On renal biopsy the major changes are in the blood vessels. Interlobular arteries show gross intimal thickening with marked reduction of the capillary lumen, which may even contain thrombi. The intimal thickening is mucinous with concentrically arranged nuclei. Afferent arterioles may show similar changes and, in addition, fibrinoid necrosis. Glomerular changes are not marked.

**Pathogenesis.** This is uncertain but may be related to a slow generalized intravascular coagulation.

**Diagnosis.** This can be made from the typical skin appearances. Biopsy will reveal intimal changes in blood vessels.

Radiology can be helpful and on renal arteriography there is a considerable reduction in the vascular phase with fairly abrupt smooth tapering of interlobular arteries. In the nephrographic phase there may be diffuse spotty lucencies and persistent filling of the arteries.

**Management.** There is no satisfactory treatment. Management can only be symptomatic and must include care to the skin and control of hypertension. Penicillamine has been used but is not of any proven value.

**Prognosis.** This is variable but if renal failure develops it is extremely poor. If acute renal failure develops there is little chance of a return of renal function. Some patients appear to remain in a stable state for many years.


## AMYLOIDOSIS

**Introduction.** Amyloidosis may be classified into several distinct groups.
   1. PRIMARY. In which there does not appear to be any underlying precipitating cause. In this group deposition is usually found in the gastrointestinal tract, heart and spleen, although the kidney is involved in approximately 35 per cent of cases.
   2. SECONDARY. Due to such conditions as chronic suppuration (e.g. osteomyelitis or bronchiectasis), tuberculosis, rheumatoid arthritis, Hodgkinson's disease, Crohn's disease, ulcerative colitis, ankylosing spondylitis or leprosy. The amyloid deposits are found in the liver, spleen, kidney and adrenals.
   3. ASSOCIATED WITH MULTIPLE MYELOMA. Occurs in approximately 15 per cent of cases and has a distribution similar to the primary form.
   4. FAMILIAL. Particularly in familial Mediterranean fever (FMF) where the incidence is approximately 50 per cent and is a major cause of death.
   5. LOCALIZED. Localized deposits of amyloid can be found in many elderly people and are probably of little consequence.

**Nature of Amyloid.** Amyloid is a protein material which is deposited extracellularly in tissues. In some cases, particularly associated with multiple myeloma and plasma cell dyscrasias, it is composed of fragments of immunoglobulins. However, in most other cases the protein is not derived from immunoglobulin and its site of production is unknown.

**Clinical Features**
   1. Proteinuria is common and there is little correlation between the amount excreted and the severity of the glomerular lesions. The proteinuria may be sufficient to produce the nephrotic syndrome.
   2. Renal failure is common and is of poor prognosis. Patients may, however, remain in a relatively stable state for some time.
   3. Sudden deterioration in renal function may be associated with renal vein thrombosis.
   4. Hypertension is variable and not common. Some patients may exhibit hypotension possibly due to cardiac involvement.
   5. Renal tubular acidosis may develop and it has been suggested that this is due to peritubular deposition.

6. Nephrogenic diabetes insipidus may also appear due to a similar mechanism to (5).
7. The kidneys are usually enlarged.

## Pathology

1. The glomeruli show patchy thickening of the capillary walls due to the deposition of eosinophilic material. These deposits enlarge so that the capillary lumina and eventually the whole tuft becomes obliterated. On electron microscopy the deposits are seen to contain fine non-branching fibrils which have been described as 'Chinese characters'. Amyloid is also found in the mesangium and this may be the earliest site of deposition.
2. The tubules may have amyloid deposited around the basement membrane.
3. The blood vessels, particularly interlobular arteries, may show infiltration in the media.
4. The interstitium is frequently affected by fibrosis, particularly in severe cases.

## Management

1. In primary amyloidosis there does not appear to be any specific therapy and so treatment is symptomatic.
2. In secondary types an attempt must be made to remove the underlying lesion. However, it must be recognized that improvement may not follow although there may be stabilization of the renal function.
3. A correct diagnosis should be established by renal biopsy.
4. If renal tubular acidosis is present it should be treated as the patient will improve symptomatically.
5. Any sudden deterioration in renal function warrants investigation for possible renal vein thrombosis.
6. Familial Mediterranean fever seems to respond to colchicine and there are hopes that the amyloidosis will concurrently improve.

**Prognosis.** Once there is biopsy-proven renal involvement the prognosis is poor. Approximately 50 per cent will develop terminal renal failure within one year.

## HENOCH–SCHÖNLEIN SYNDROME (ANAPHYLACTOID PURPURA)

**Introduction.** This is a syndrome characterized by a purpuric skin lesion involving the arms, legs, buttocks and lower back, associated with:

1. Joint pain and swelling.
2. Gastrointestinal symptoms of colic, vomiting and blood loss.
3. Glomerulonephritis.

The frequency and severity and combination of these clinical manifestations is variable.

**Aetiology.** Probably of allergic origin and bacterial infections, food, insect bites and drugs have been implicated.

**Pathogenesis.** The various clinical manifestations are due to antigen—antibody complexes becoming deposited in blood vessels producing a vasculitis and inflammatory response.

**Clinical Features**
1. The skin manifestations usually appear first and may have been preceded by an infective illness. There may be simultaneous joint and gastrointestinal involvement.
2. Renal manifestations usually appear within 4 weeks of the purpura. It may vary from asymptomatic proteinuria, gross or microscopic haematuria, acute nephritis, nephrotic syndrome to acute renal failure.
3. Children are more commonly affected than adults, and males more than females.
4. Renal involvement appears to be more severe in adults.

**Pathology.** The renal biopsy appearances are variable and depend to some extent on the severity of the syndrome. The glomeruli may show:
1. Focal and segmental proliferation with or without small crescents.
2. A mild diffuse proliferative lesion.
3. A proliferation associated with many large circumferential crescents.

In severe lesions interlobular arteries and afferent arterioles may show inflammatory necrotizing changes, and the interstitium extensive tubular damage and inflammatory infiltrate.

**Management.** Depends to a large extent on the severity of the illness. In children the majority make a very satisfactory recovery although a number will have persistent urinary abnormalities such as mild proteinuria and microscopical haematuria. In patients with severe renal involvement steroids with or without immunosuppression may be of value.

**Prognosis.** The skin, joint and gastrointestinal manifestations are usually self-limiting. In patients with focal and segmental glomerulonephritis on biopsy the prognosis is good, whereas those with many circumferential crescents have a poor prognosis. Children have a good prognosis, but approximately 50 per cent of adults will progress to renal failure.

## DIABETES MELLITUS

**Introduction.** The kidney may be involved in several ways in a patient who has diabetes mellitus — diabetic glomerulosclerosis, pyelonephritis, papillary necrosis and vascular changes.

### Diabetic Glomerulosclerosis
**Pathology.** There are four well recognized glomerular lesions.
1. Nodular glomerulosclerosis (Kimmelstiel—Wilson lesion) where

there are homogeneous, eosinophilic areas situated in the central part of lobules, particularly towards the periphery of the tuft. There may be several such nodules, usually of different size within a glomerulus.
2. Diffuse glomerulosclerosis in which there is widespread diffuse increase in the mesangial regions, associated with capillary wall thickening. The diffuse lesion is more common than the nodular.
3. Fibrin cap. This is an accumulation of eosinophilic material in the concavity of a peripheral capillary loop.
4. Capsular drop. This is a localized eosinophilic mass on Bowman's capsule.

Arteries and arterioles frequently show sclerosis.

### Clinical Features
1. The incidence of glomerular lesions increases with age and the duration of diabetes.
2. It is probably more common in poorly controlled diabetics but this is by no means certain.
3. Proteinuria is the most common clinical manifestation. This may proceed to the nephrotic syndrome.
4. Hypertension is common.
5. Nephropathy is frequently accompanied by retinopathy and neuropathy.
6. Following the development of nephrotic syndrome progression to renal failure is common and fairly rapid, the mean time to end-stage renal failure being approximately 3 years.

### Management
1. Good diabetic control should be achieved.
2. The nephrotic syndrome should be treated with diuretics but a careful watch needs to be made of the insulin requirements as these are likely to be altered.
3. Hypertension must be controlled.
4. Renal failure should be treated by conventional means.
5. Haemodialysis is associated with a poor survival and it may be that continuous ambulatory peritoneal dialysis is of more value. Transplantation is attended by many complications although success has been reported from some centres.

## GOUT

**Introduction.** Gout is a syndrome caused by the deposition of uric acid crystals in tissues. These deposits occur in joints, subcutaneous tissues and soft tissues. The raised plasma uric acid concentration can be either:
1. PRIMARY, due to a defect in intermediary purine metabolism, or
2. SECONDARY, due to either overproduction of urates as in myeloproliferative diseases (particularly when treatment is commenced)

or in severe chronic renal failure where excretion of urates is impaired.

**Renal Involvement**
1. INTERSTITIAL NEPHRITIS. This results from uric acid crystal deposition with subsequent inflammatory changes. It most commonly occurs in the medulla.
2. PYELONEPHRITIS. Infection is frequently superimposed on the interstitial nephritis and may result in considerable destruction of tissue.
3. CALCULI. Uric acid stones occur in approximately 15–20 per cent of patients with primary gout, and 40 per cent of those with secondary gout. The stones are radiolucent and therefore not seen on X-ray unless they also contain calcium.
4. ACUTE RENAL FAILURE. This may develop in secondary gout particularly at the beginning of treatment of myeloproliferative disorders. Uric acid crystals form in the tubules and produce an obstructive uropathy. Prophylactic treatment with bicarbonate and a high fluid intake should be undertaken, where such a situation is likely to develop.
5. CHRONIC RENAL FAILURE. Can result from the interstitial nephritis, infection or the increased incidence of hypertension. Chronic renal failure itself will produce an elevation in plasma uric acid concentration but this rarely leads to gouty symptoms.

**Management**
1. PRIMARY GOUT. Urate formation can be reduced by the xanthine oxidase inhibitor (Allopurinol).
2. URIC ACID STONES. In addition to Allopurinol a high urine flow rate should be maintained. Uric acid is poorly soluble at pH 6 or less and thus an alkaline urine should be maintained. This may require considerable bicarbonate supplements which may be difficult for the patient.
3. ACUTE RENAL FAILURE. Most likely to occur early in the cytotoxic treatment of myeloproliferative disorders. In the established case the management is no different from other cases (*see* Chapter 7). It may be prevented by establishing a high flow rate of alkaline urine prior to starting cytotoxic therapy.
4. CHRONIC RENAL FAILURE. Treated in a conventional way (*see* Chapter 8).
5. HYPERTENSION. This frequently complicates gout. Treatment is along conventional lines but it must be remembered that thiazides may potentiate gout.
6. INFECTION. Commonly occurs in gout but may be difficult to diagnose due to the frequently occurring sterile pyuria. As

infections may produce sudden and severe deterioration in renal function they must be treated promptly.

## SARCOIDOSIS

Renal involvement in sarcoidosis may occur due to the following:
1. SARCOID GRANULOMA infiltrating the kidney but this rarely is sufficient to impair renal function.
2. INTERSTITIAL NEPHRITIS resulting from calcium deposition or sarcoid granulomata.
3. NEPHROCALCINOSIS due to the hypercalcaemia.
4. CALCULI which are frequently multiple and bilateral.
5. GLOMERULONEPHRITIS may rarely occur. The reported cases have all had a membranous appearance and have been shown to contain immunoglobulins. The pathogenesis is unknown.

Management is by controlling the underlying sarcoidosis and dealing with the renal complications as and when they develop. Hypercalcaemia and nephrocalcinosis should be treated by steroids.

## SUBACUTE BACTERIAL ENDOCARDITIS

Bacterial endocarditis may be complicated by renal involvement in the following ways:
1. Focal glomerulonephritis which may present as an acute nephritis or be detected by routine urinalysis. This occurs in about 50 per cent of patients with subacute bacterial endocarditis.
2. Diffuse proliferative glomerulonephritis presenting as an acute nephritis. The severity of this complication is variable but acute renal failure has been reported. Both forms of glomerulonephritis are thought to be due to the deposition of antigen–antibody complexes derived from the endocardial lesions.
3. Renal infarcts due to obstruction of arcuate or large interlobular arteries by embolic material from the endocardium. These are frequently asymptomatic but may be associated with macroscopic haematuria.

The management is aimed primarily at the cardiac lesion and consists of appropriate antibiotic therapy for at least 6 weeks. Repeated blood culture may be necessary to determine the underlying organism. The progress of the valvular lesion can be followed by echocardiography. If renal failure develops it is managed along conventional lines (*see* Chapters 7 and 8).

# Chapter 11

# URINARY TRACT INFECTIONS

Introduction – Definition of terminology – Causal organisms – Normal defence mechanisms – Route of infection – Predisposing factors – Asymptomatic infections (covert bacteriuria) – Symptomatic infections – Vesico-ureteric reflux – Renal tuberculosis

## INTRODUCTION

Urinary tract infection is important because of its frequency and its association with renal failure. The subject is complicated by terminology which is not standardized and which, at first, appears confusing. The reason for this difficulty is mainly due to the increasing awareness that infection may present clinically in several ways and that in certain conditions, such as 'chronic pyelonephritis', identical end-stage appearances may be produced by widely differing pathological processes.

In females the incidence of urinary tract infection increases with age and some 5 per cent of adult women will, at some time, develop infection. In males there is a high incidence in the neonatal period, a low incidence in childhood and adult life, and a further increase with advancing years. Urinary tract infection accounts for about 1–2 per cent of consultation in general practice. End-stage renal failure as a result of urinary tract infection is the cause in 20 per cent of patients requiring long-term haemodialysis.

## DEFINITION OF TERMINOLOGY

It is of utmost importance to understand and to employ correct terminology. In addition, it is of value to refrain from jumping to conclusions regarding diagnosis until the appropriate diagnostic criteria are satisfied.

*Urinary Tract Infection*: The presence of micro-organisms in the urinary tract with or without signs or symptoms of inflammation.

*Bacteriuria*: This is the presence of bacteria in the urine. It is considered significant if the numbers of bacteria exceed 100 000/ml in a properly collected specimen examined correctly. The presence of bacteria may be accompanied by clinical symptoms or may be asymptomatic (covert bacteria).

*Pyuria*: This is the presence of pus cells in the urine and is always considered significant. It may be associated with bacteria but in certain circumstances there are no bacteria identifiable and it is designated as sterile pyuria.

*Dysuria*: This is a symptom of pain or discomfort in the urethra or meatal area on micturition.

*Frequency and Polyuria*: These terms are frequently used synonymously but they must not be confused. Frequency refers to frequent emptying of the bladder while polyuria indicates the passage of large amounts of urine.

*Bacterial Cystitis*: A syndrome of dysuria and frequency accompanied by bacteriuria, pyuria and sometimes haematuria.

*Abacterial Cystitis* (*urethral syndrome*): A syndrome of dysuria and frequency in the absence of bacteriuria.

*Pyelonephritis*: Inflammation within the substance of the kidney. Acute bacterial pyelonephritis is a syndrome consisting of loin pain, tenderness and pyrexia accompanied by bacteriuria, pyuria and sometimes haematuria. Chronic pyelonephritis is a term which has fallen into disrepute due to misusage and the term 'chronic interstitial nephritis' is to be preferred. This is a chronic inflammatory disease affecting the interstitium and tubules which leads to scarring due to progressive shrinkage from interstitial fibrosis. It may be produced by many causes, including bacterial infection, but in many instances the aetiology is unknown.

## CAUSAL ORGANISMS

The organisms responsible for urinary tract infection are:

*Escherichia coli* – this is the most common bacteria isolated and accounts for infection in approximately 80 per cent of cases. In most patients the organism will also be present as normal bowel flora.

*Klebsiella, Proteus, Pseudomonas* are more commonly isolated from patients with structural abnormalities of the urinary tract or following instrumentation, catheterization or after antibiotic therapy.

*Staphylococcus aureus* – this rarely produces urinary tract infection and if present it should be isolated in significant numbers from repeated specimens before being considered pathological. If thought to be significant careful search should be made to determine the primary source of the infection, e.g. abscess or osteomyelitis. *Staphylococcus albus* infections account for 20 per cent of infections in sexually active women.

*Mycobacterium tuberculosis* – this should always be considered when pyuria is present but no significant bacterial growth obtained on culture. Early morning samples of urine (EMU) on three occasions should be examined.

Fungi (*Candida albicans*) seldom produce infection in normal patients but may become a problem in immunosuppressed patients (e.g. patients with renal transplants).

## NORMAL DEFENCE MECHANISMS

Urine provides a satisfactory growth medium for bacteria but the normal person has several defence mechanisms to prevent infections.

1. MECHANICAL. The flow of urine is such that bacteria tend to be washed out by voiding and the number of bacteria in the bladder is constantly being diluted by the flow of urine from the kidneys. The number of organisms in the bladder therefore depends upon

the urine flow rate, the completeness of emptying on micturition and the rate of bacterial multiplication. The route of the ureter through the bladder muscle is such that on bladder contraction at micturition the ureteric orifice is closed thereby preventing the flow of urine from bladder to ureter.

2. MUCOSAL. The bladder mucosa secretes IgA which is bactericidal. This is only active close to the mucosa and if there is incomplete bladder emptying there may be an amount of residual urine with no effective cidal action where bacteria can multiply. Prostatic and urethral secretions also contain substances which are bactericidal or bacteriostatic. Organisms which gain access to the bladder have villi which provide considerable adherence to the urothelium. Secretory IgA, from the urethra, inhibits the adhering ability of the organisms thereby causing their washout during micturition.

## ROUTE OF INFECTION

Infection may gain access to the urinary tract from the blood or from ascent of perineal organisms.

1. HAEMATOGENOUS. This is rare apart from infections in neonates, in severe septicaemia and in tuberculous infections.

2. ASCENDING INFECTION. Urinary tract infection is most commonly due to organisms which are present in the patient's bowel flora. In the female, introital colonization precedes bladder invasion. The bowel organisms which gain access to the renal tract have villi which give considerable adherence to the urothelium thereby providing protection from the mechanical effect of micturition and washing. Infection in the female is more common than in the male because of (*a*) the short female urethra, (*b*) the turbulent flow in the female urethra allows ascent of organisms against the stream at micturition, (*c*) the lack of prostatic secretions which are bacteriostatic, and (*d*) the trauma associated with coitus and parturition. Urethral secretions contain IgA which should reduce the ability of organisms to adhere to the urothelium and if the secretory IgA is deficient then organisms will gain access more easily. Infection can also be introduced by instrumentation such as at catheterization or cystoscopy.

Organisms which gain access to the bladder will normally be removed by micturition and the action of IgA. However, if bladder emptying is incomplete the organisms will have the opportunity to multiply, and bladder wall inflammation (cystitis) will occur. If the inflammation is severe it may interfere with the normal valve action of the vesico-ureteric junction. In this way urine may reflux into the ureter on micturition. Ascent of infection to the kidneys is then possible. Ascent may be enhanced by the production, by some bacteria, of 'toxins' which inhibit urethral peristalsis.

The ascent of organisms from the bladder to the kidney is dependent on the severity of reflux and there is a close association between reflux and renal scarring. Once bacteria reach the kidney they can gain access to the medulla where they multiply due to (*a*) the medullary high osmolality inhibiting leucocyte mobilization, (*b*) the high osmolality allowing the development of L forms, and (*c*) the high ammonia concentration inhibiting the effect of complement. It is likely that the bacteria which gain access to the kidney are in some way 'selected' as *E. coli* isolated from patients with kidney infections are less susceptible to the cidal effect of serum than organisms isolated from infections localized to the bladder.

## PREDISPOSING FACTORS

There are certain factors which predispose to infection in the renal tract.

1. In the female, the short urethra (*vide supra*).
2. Instrumentation. Catheterization must be aseptically performed and any indwelling catheter must be carefully maintained to prevent infection.
3. Structural abnormalities. Any structural abnormality confers an increased susceptibility to infection and this is greatly increased if any stasis is present. Patients with polycystic disease and bladder diverticula are therefore prone to infection.
4. Pregnancy. Infection occurs in about 5 per cent of pregnant patients. This is due to the effect of oestrogens on the muscle of the renal tract and the fact that there tends to be dilatation of the upper tract with relative stasis.
5. Calculi. Not only do these increase the liability to infection, they make eradication virtually impossible. Infection in the presence of calculi may well change the composition of the stone (*see* Chapter 12, p. 140).
6. Analgesic nephropathy. There is damage to the renal papillae and this renders the medulla more susceptible to infection.
7. Obstruction. Interference with the mechanical effect of urine flow increases the risk of infection. This probably accounts for the increasing incidence of infection in older men who develop obstruction from prostatic hypertrophy.
8. Diabetes mellitus. The diabetic urine provides an excellent culture medium and, in addition, there may be medullary damage and interference with micturition from neuropathy.
9. Spinal injuries. If there is spinal cord damage motor and sensory fibres may be affected resulting in a neurogenic bladder, with incomplete emptying and stasis. In addition many of these patients will have indwelling catheters.

10. Vesico-ureteric reflux. This is probably the result of infection. Renal scarring correlates with the degree of reflux and liability to damage is greatest in the first four years of life.

## ASYMPTOMATIC INFECTIONS (COVERT BACTERIURIA)

The incidence of asymptomatic bacteriuria varies with age and sex. In schoolgirls the incidence is just less than 2 per cent but with age there is a steady increase to approximately 6 per cent in females aged over 60. In schoolboys the incidence is less than 0·2 per cent and this does not increase until old age. In females the incidence is greater in married than single and greater in parous than nulliparous patients.

Investigation of schoolgirls with asymptomatic bacteriuria reveals a high incidence of urinary tract abnormalities on i.v.p.

| | |
|---|---|
| Bladder wall thickening and irregularity | 5 per cent |
| Reflux | 15 per cent |
| Reflux and renal scarring | 25 per cent |

Scars are more common in the upper than the lower pole and are rare in the middle calyceal system. They are commonly associated with reflux and do not appear to develop after the age of 5 years.

### Management

1. Investigate the structure of the urinary tract by i.v.p. and micturating cystogram in children of either sex and in adult males.
2. There is no need to treat except in particular circumstances (*see* 3). Spontaneous cure occurs in 10 per cent of patients. Antibiotic treatment will render the urine sterile in more than 90 per cent of cases but 30 per cent will recur and those who become reinfected are likely to be symptomatic.
3. The infection should be treated in:
   a. Early childhood.
   b. Patients with impaired immunity.
   c. Pregnancy because spontaneous cure does not appear to occur and 40 per cent are likely to develop pyelonephritis.

In such patients treatment should be carried out with the most appropriate antibiotic and then follow-up to ensure continuing sterility of the urine.

## SYMPTOMATIC INFECTIONS

Symptomatic infections occur in infants, particularly females under 2 years who are at risk from perineal soiling. In adult females there is an increased incidence concurrent with sexual activity and at late middle age when gynaecological problems such as prolapse and vaginitis become more common. In males the incidence is low until later in life when prostatic obstruction becomes common.

The symptoms of infection confined to the bladder are frequency and dysuria with little constitutional upset. In acute upper tract infections there is fever, dysuria, urgency and frequency associated with haematuria, loin pain, abdominal pain and kidney tenderness. In chronic upper tract infections there is low back pain, nocturia, fatigability, weight loss and anorexia. While symptoms may help to localize infections they are only a guide and are not reliable. It must be remembered that urinary tract infections can be remarkably asymptomatic.

The diagnosis is made by quantitative urine culture with the finding of greater than $10^5$ organisms/ml urine. However, significant infection may be present if a pure growth of bacteria is obtained from urine which also contained pus cells. Some infections with low bacterial counts are due to high urine flow rates, frequent micturition and bacteria adhering to pus cells, thus giving false low counts.

Investigation must include culture of urine collected under satisfactory conditions. It is not necessary to carry out an i.v.p. in all patients and this should be reserved for:

1. Males of all ages.
2. Females up to the age of puberty whether symptomatic or not.
3. Adult females with a history of more than three symptomatic episodes or a history of childhood infections.

In chronic pyelonephritis the i.v.p. shows small irregularly contracted kidneys with calyceal clubbing and overlying cortical contraction.

## Management

1. Obtain satisfactory urine culture, twice if possible.
2. Investigate further if indicated.
3. High fluid intake to achieve a high urine flow rate.
4. Teach patients perineal hygiene.
5. Antibiotic therapy should aim to achieve an adequate urinary concentration of the antibiotic to which the infecting bacteria is sensitive. The vast majority of infections are due to *E. coli* and will be sensitive to ampicillin, cephalosporins, trimethoprim and co-trimoxazole. Hospital-acquired infections are less likely to be susceptible to ampicillin. Klebsiella, Proteus and Pseudomonas infections are more likely to require gentamicin, tobramycin or carbenicillin. The length of therapy must be adequate and, although the trend is towards shorter courses, at least 7 days is required in most patients.
6. Although a 7-day course of an appropriate antibiotic will cure 80 per cent or more some 60 per cent will have a recurrence within the subsequent 12 months. Recurrence is due to either relapse or reinfection.
   Relapse commonly occurs shortly after treatment, 85 per cent within the first month. The causes of relapse are: wrong choice

of antibiotic; inadequate duration of therapy; non-compliance; emergence of resistant strain; development of L forms; urolithiasis.

Treatment of relapses is by ensuring an adequate course of appropriate antibiotic.

Reinfection accounts for 80 per cent of recurrent infections, the majority appearing some 1–5 months after a treated infection. Reinfection is most common where there is a failure of the normal defence mechanisms or the presence of some structural abnormality. Reinfection can be treated by the patient inoculating a dip-slide for culture and then taking a 7-day course of an appropriate antibiotic. In this way prompt treatment can take place with adequate bacteriological control.

7. Prophylactic therapy can be used for patients who have frequent recurrences, i.e. greater than 4 yearly. The most appropriate suppressive drugs are:

| Nitrofurantoin | 50 mg |
| Cephalexin | 125 mg |
| Co-trimoxazole | 1 tab |
| Methenamine | 1 g |

and they should be taken at night.

Methenamine in acid urine is hydrolysed to form formaldehyde; thus to be effective the urine must be acid and so ammonium chloride may be required. If the renal function is impaired there may be accumulation of mandelic acid and so it should not be used if the creatinine clearance is less than 50 ml/min.

8. If recurrences frequently follow coitus a satisfactory response may be obtained by a simple regime of bladder emptying and a single dose of an antibiotic after intercourse.

9. Surgery can be of value in the relief of obstruction, the removal of stones and the removal of an infected non-functioning kidney.


## VESICO-URETERIC REFLUX

Vesico-ureteric reflux occurs when the integrity of the vesico-ureteric junction is destroyed so that on bladder contraction urine can flow from the bladder back up into the ureter. The extent of the reflux can be graded on a micturating cystogram.

Grade I:   flow into ureter but not as far as the kidney.

Grade II:  flow as far as the kidney but no calyceal distension.

Grade III: flow reaching the kidney and causing calyceal distension.

There is a close association between reflux and renal scarring, 85 per cent of scarred kidneys have reflux. There also appears to be a familial incidence of reflux. It is not present in normal patients but occurs in 20 per cent of patients with asymptomatic bacteriuria and 35 per cent of patients with symptomatic infections.

The management of reflux is difficult to determine as there have been no satisfactory large-scale controlled studies to evaluate the role of surgery. Mild reflux, grades I and II, usually clear spontaneously. In severe reflux, grade III, surgery can correct the abnormality and reduce the incidence of symptomatic infections. The aim of surgery is to prevent the development of renal scarring. As scars do not seem to develop after the age of 5 years surgery needs to be considered in pre-school children. In children in whom reflux stops spontaneously, after conservative therapy, or after surgery, 85 per cent have satisfactory kidney growth while those with continual reflux only 60 per cent grow. The progression to chronic renal failure is due to back pressure on the kidneys from severe reflux.

The child who develops scars is unlikely to develop further renal damage provided infection is controlled, the blood pressure remains normal and there is no obstructive uropathy. Upper pole scars, however, increase the incidence of hypertension in pregnancy and during oral contraceptive therapy.

## RENAL TUBERCULOSIS

Tuberculous infection of the renal tract is not rare but is frequently forgotten. It should be considered in all patients who are found to have a sterile pyuria.

**Pathogenesis.** Renal tuberculosis is due to infection with *Mycobacterium tuberculosis*. The infection is blood-borne and generally the cortex is initially affected and most cases are bilateral. The papillae become involved and caseous lesions develop with subsequent ulceration and calcification. Infection spreads down the renal tract and strictures of the ureters, particularly at the vesico-ureteric junction are common. Bladder involvement gives rise to contraction and consequent diminution in capacity. In male patients the epididymis may become infected and the caseous lesions may form a chronic discharging sinus. Thus tuberculosis may involve the whole of the renal tract.

**Clinical Features.** There may be a surprising lack of symptoms even in severely involved cases. The most common symptoms are fever, dysuria, frequency, nocturia, back pain, loin pain, haematuria and weight loss.

Routine urine culture will reveal a sterile pyuria and to establish a diagnosis early morning urine (EMU) samples should be examined for *Mycobacterium tuberculosis*. Isolation and culture may be difficult and it is advisable to examine at least three EMU samples.

The i.v.p. may show the following features: calcified caseous lesions in the papillae; gross destruction of pelvicalyceal system; hydronephrosis; ureteric obstruction; contracted bladder; evidence of calcification in caseous material at any point in renal tract.

Diagnosis of renal tuberculosis depends to a large extent on remembering the possibility of tuberculous infection and carefully searching for the causative organism.

**Management**

1. Establish accurate diagnosis.
2. Treat with appropriate antituberculous drugs for at least 6 months. Many patients have impaired renal function at the time of diagnosis and so the dosage of the drugs may need to be modified (*see* Chapter 15).
3. After treatment has been started there may be considerable oedema of the lesions and this may produce an increased obstruction. Sequential renogram studies provides a useful means of monitoring this potential hazard.
4. During healing there may be the development of fibrosis with stricture formation in the ureter and/or urethra. Steroid therapy may alleviate this problem but there is controversy on this point.
5. Surgery may be required to relieve obstruction of the ureter or urethra, or to remove a non-functioning kidney. Surgery may also be of value in enlarging a severely constricted bladder. In severe obstructive cases nephrostomy may prove useful in decompressing a kidney and preserving renal function.
6. In cases progressing to transplantation there is a need for careful evaluation of the lower urinary tract to ensure that there is no bladder or urethral involvement which would interfere with normal micturition.

# Chapter 12

# RENAL CALCULI, NEPHROCALCINOSIS AND HYPERCALCIURIA

Introduction – Nephrocalcinosis – Nephrolithiasis – Hypercalciuria

## INTRODUCTION

Calcification in the kidneys and urinary tract can be due to a wide variety of causes. The calcification may be diffuse or localized, may be due to metabolic diseases or infections and may, depending on the aetiology, occur at any age.

The incidence of renal stone disease appears to be increasing while that of bladder stone disease is decreasing. There are widespread geographical differences in the pattern of stone disease, renal stones being more common in industrial 'westernized' countries while bladder stones are more common, particularly in boys, in poorer agricultural economies. It is likely that changes in dietary habits are responsible for this changing pattern.

The major conditions causing calcification in the kidneys and renal tract can be considered as:
1. Nephrocalcinosis.
2. Nephrolithiasis.
3. Infections, particularly tuberculosis.
4. Medullary cystic disease.
5. Cortical necrosis and renal infarction.
6. Tumours.
7. Bladder stone disease.

## NEPHROCALCINOSIS

This is a diffuse deposition of calcium in the substance of the kidney, most commonly in the papillae of the medulla. It does not include localized areas of calcium deposition as is frequently seen in tuberculosis, as a sequelae to necrosis or infarct or associated with certain tumours. It may arise from:
1. A generalized renal disorder.
2. The deposition of calcium as carbonate or phosphate from hypercalcaemia, hypercalciuria, acid/base disorders or hyperphosphaturia.
3. Congenital oxalosis.

The symptoms of nephrocalcinosis are usually mild and are usually associated with:
1. Symptoms of the underlying disease.
2. Subsequent stone formation.

3. Superadded infection.
4. Induced tubular defect, e.g. polyuria.

The diagnosis of nephrocalcinosis is difficult. Radiological evidence is not present until late in the disease but the findings are of small diffuse opacities predominantly in the papillae. Renal biopsy can be helpful but as the deposits are in the medulla it is frequently necessary to proceed to open biopsy and this is seldom justified.

The causes of nephrocalcinosis are:

| | |
|---|---|
| Hypercalcaemia | Hyperparathyroidism |
| | Myelomatosis |
| Hypercalciuria | Excess vitamin D therapy |
| | Milk alkali syndrome |
| | Idiopathic hypercalciuria |
| | Sarcoidosis |
| | Carcinomatosis |
| | Immobilization |
| Alkaline urine | Alkalosis |
| | Renal tubular acidosis |
| Oxalosis | Primary |
| | Secondary |

The management of nephrocalcinosis is aimed at the underlying condition, prompt treatment of any infection and correction of any abnormal electrolyte pattern with appropriate supplements.

## NEPHROLITHIASIS

**Introduction.** Renal stone disease is due to the formation in the urine of crystal aggregates of urinary salts or acids. The crystals may form in the collecting ducts or in the calyceal system and they grow by a process of precipitation and crystallization, to form stones.

The various types of renal stone are:

| *Type* | *Cause* |
|---|---|
| Calcium oxalate | Hypercalciuria |
| and calcium phosphate | Hyperparathyroidism |
| | Hypercalcaemia |
| | Hyperuricosuria |
| | Many unknown |
| Calcium oxalate | Hyperoxaluria |
| | Oxalosis |
| Uric acid | Persistently acid urine |
| | Hyperuricaemia |
| | Myeloproliferative diseases |
| Cystine | Cystinuria |
| Xanthine | Xanthinuria |

Stone analysis can be helpful in determining the underlying cause of the renal stone disease but it should be remembered that the presence of a stone predisposes the patient to urinary tract infection. This may lead to the deposition of magnesium ammonium phosphate on the already present stone thus making difficult the interpretation of stone analysis data. However, the absence of magnesium probably means that infection is not present.

**Clinical Features.** The clinical features of calculi are (1) those caused by the underlying disease and (2) those related to the presence of the foreign body within the kidney or urinary tract.

The symptoms due to the presence of a stone in the renal tract are:
1. In the renal pelvis – a dull aching loin pain with or without episodes of colic.
2. Passage down ureter – intense colic, frequently of sudden onset and radiating to the groin.
3. In the bladder – suprapubic and perineal discomfort associated with frequency and dysuria.

The symptoms are dependent upon the size of the stone but it is remarkable that even large stones can be asymptomatic. Commonly patients only become symptomatic when the stone moves within the renal tract thus precipitating an episode of colic.

At presentation the site of the stone is:

| | |
|---|---|
| Bladder | 15 per cent |
| Ureter | 20 per cent |
| Kidney | 25 per cent |
| Passed spontaneously | 40 per cent |

Dysuria and frequency are common, especially if infection is present. Macroscopic haematuria occurs episodically and is frequently related to stone movement; microscopic haematuria is often present even in asymptomatic patients. The continued presence of white cells in the urine in the absence of any infection should raise the possibility of stone disease.

**Pathogenesis.** Stones develop by the formation of crystals of salts or acids which are present in urine. The crystals aggregate and grow due to the continued apposition of more salt or acid from the urine. The initial formation of the crystal may be due to:
1. The concentration of salt or acid exceeding that of the solubility of the salt or acid thereby resulting in crystal formation. Urine may be supersaturated but a crystal nidus will form when the concentration exceeds a certain limit of stability.
2. A reduction in inhibitors of crystal formation. Certain substances such as pyrophosphate and glycosaminoglycans have an inhibitory effect with respect to crystal growth and so a diminution in the concentration of these agents will allow crystal formation to occur at a lower salt concentration.

3.  Changes in urine pH. The pH of the urine can affect the solubility of salts. A change in urine pH such as in renal tubular acidosis will lead to an increased probability of crystallization and subsequent crystal growth.

**Calcium Stone Disease.** Calcium stones consist of calcium oxalate, calcium oxalate and calcium phosphate, and uncommonly calcium phosphate by itself. Factors leading to the formation of calcium containing stones are:
1.  Hypercalciuria.
2.  Hyperoxaluria.
3.  Increased urine pH.
4.  Diminished urine volume.
5.  Diminished urinary glycosaminoglycans.
6.  Hyperuricosuria.

The major causes of calcium stone disease are:
1.  IDIOPATHIC. The majority of patients with calcium stone disease do not appear to have any underlying cause. In some there is an increased intestinal absorption of calcium leading to hypercalciuria, less commonly there appears to be a renal 'leak' of calcium giving rise to hypercalciuria. The factors responsible for these abnormalities are unknown.

    The majority of patients are males and there is a peak incidence in middle age. There is frequently a strong family history but the mode of inheritance is unknown. It is most likely polygenic with a reduced risk in females.

    The clinical course is very variable. It commonly starts in young adult life and some patients exhibit repeated stone formation while others appear to have long periods of remission.

    Management consists of:
    a.  Investigation to exclude secondary causes of calcium stones.
    b.  Dietary advice to reduce the urine calcium and oxalate concentrations, i.e. low calcium, low oxalate, high fluid intake.
    c.  Thiazide diuretics – the mode of action is to reduce urinary calcium excretion although the means by which this is achieved is unknown. Side effects include hypokalaemia and mild hypercalcaemia.
    d.  Sodium cellulose phosphate – this is a non-absorbable ion exchange resin with a high affinity for calcium. Thus there is intestinal trapping of calcium with a consequent reduction in absorption.
    e.  Orthophosphate – this promotes the urinary excretion of pyrophosphate and so reduces the tendency to crystal formation. The side effects include soft tissue calcification and bone loss.
    f.  Diphosphonates – good theoretically but probably produce osteomalacia.

Specific therapy is not available and the drugs listed all have to be used on a long-term basis. The condition has a very variable natural history and so therapy is not indicated unless the patient is a recurrent stone former and in such instances careful follow-up is essential.

2.  HYPERPARATHYROIDISM. This is more common in females and accounts for something less than 10 per cent of recurrent calcium stone formers. The factors which precipitate stone formation in patients with hyperparathyroidism are:

*a.*  Hypercalciuria due to increased intestinal absorption and bone reabsorption.

*b.*  High urine pH due to the inhibition of bicarbonate reabsorption by PTH.

The diagnosis of hyperparathyroidism depends on the clinical findings of nephrolithiasis, bone disease and peptic ulcer disease associated with hypercalcaemia, hypercalciuria and a raised plasma PTH concentration. Patients may also complain of headache, muscle weakness, fatigability, polyuria and thirst. In most patients, however, many of these features will be absent and a correct diagnosis will only be achieved by careful and often repeated investigation.

Management is by careful assessment and subsequent parathyroidectomy. Removal of the abnormal parathyroid tissue stops active stone formation and frequently existing stones will, with time, break up and be passed spontaneously.

3.  RENAL TUBULAR ACIDOSIS. Stones are associated with primary RTA of the distal type (Type 1) (*see* Chapter 13, p. 152) and secondary forms (*see* Chapter 14, p. 154).

4.  MEDULLARY SPONGE KIDNEY. *See* Chapter 13, p. 147.

5.  HYPERCALCIURIA. Conditions associated with increased urinary calcium excretion which may result in the formation of stone:

 Vitamin D intoxication.
 Sarcoidosis.
 Milk-alkali syndrome.
 Prolonged immobilization.
 Cushing's syndrome and prolonged steroid therapy.
 Paget's disease.
 Carcinomatosis.

6.  HYPERURICOSURIA. Increased urinary uric acid excretion can lead to the formation of calcium stones in the absence of hypercalciuria. The increased uric acid is probably the result of a high purine diet. The mode of action is probably by diminishing the inhibitory effect of glycosaminoglycans on crystal formation. Management is by dietary reduction of purines and possibly allopurinol.

The management of patients with calcium stone disease is

by treatment of the underlying condition, the maintenance of a high fluid intake, frequent monitoring for infection and stone removal if obstruction occurs.

**Infected Stone Disease.** The stones which form secondary to urinary tract infection consist of magnesium ammonium phosphate and variable amounts of calcium phosphate. They are frequently bilateral and are situated in the renal pelvis where they may grow to fill the whole pelvis thereby forming a staghorn calculus. The factors which lead to the formation of these stones are a high urinary ammonia concentration and a high urine pH. The high ammonia concentration is due to the ability of certain bacteria to split urea to ammonia and carbon dioxide.

Infected stone disease is common in situations of urinary stasis and in patients with structural abnormalities. Any factor leading to urinary tract infection such as analgesic abuse, instrumentation, obstructive uropathy or urinary tract surgery may predispose to subsequent stone formation. In addition the presence of any stone, no matter of what type, may be complicated by superadded infection with a consequent change in the composition of the stone. The presence of magnesium in the stone is highly suggestive of an element of infection being present.

Management consists of:

1. Determining the size and site of the stones present in the urinary tract.
2. Assessing the degree of renal impairment.
3. The surgical removal of the stone or stones and the correction of any underlying abnormality such as obstruction or structural abnormality.
4. The sterilization of the urine with the most appropriate antibiotic regimen.
5. The long-term follow-up of the patient to ensure the urine remains sterile.
6. Careful repeated examination of the urinary tract to detect the development of any further stones.

**Uric Acid Stone Disease.** Uric acid stones form when there is a high urinary uric acid concentration and/or a persistently low urinary pH. High urinary uric acid concentration can be due to a high dietary purine intake or gout. Uric acid is poorly soluble in acid urine and crystals are likely to form if the urine is persistently below pH 6. A persistently low urinary pH is found in failure of adequate renal ammonium production, an increased dietary acid or in ileostomy patients from the persistent intestinal loss of alkaline gut contents. Thus uric acid stones are found in patients with:

1. Gout.
2. Myeloproliferative disorders.
3. High dietary purine intake.
4. Uricosuric drug treatment.

5.  Ileostomy.
6.  Dehydration.
7.  Increased dietary acid from high animal protein intake.

Uric acid stones are radiolucent and so will not be seen on X-ray unless they also contain calcium. They are more common in males and there appears to be some genetic predisposition as a family history is commonly present. In other respects the clinical features do not differ from patients with other types of stones.

Management is by:

1.  Achieving a urine volume of greater than 2 l daily which requires an oral intake of about 3 l daily.
2.  Maintaining a urine persistently in excess of pH 6 with alkali, normally this requires 10–20 g sodium bicarbonate daily and many patients find this impossible.
3.  Allopurinol if hyperuricaemia or hyperuricosuria is present.

**Cystine Stone Disease.** This is caused by an autosomal recessive condition characterized by abnormal tubular handling of cystine, ornithine, arginine and lysine (cystinuria). Cystine, being the least soluble of these amino acids, forms crystals when the urine concentration is high (*see* Chapter 13, p. 150).

**Hyperoxaluria.** Hyperoxaluria occurs as a primary condition which is rare and is autosomal recessive. There is a metabolic defect resulting in the accumulation of glyoxylate which is a precursor of oxalate. The condition becomes manifest in childhood and usually presents with symptoms of renal calculi. There is nephrolithiasis, nephrocalcinosis and widespread tissue deposition of oxalate. Calcium oxalate stones are markedly radio-opaque. The prognosis is poor and death is usually due to chronic renal failure from nephrolithiasis, urinary tract infection and obstruction.

Secondary hyperoxaluria has been reported in:

Intestinal disease.
Ileal resection.
Intestinal bypass operation.
Pyridoxine deficiency.
Methoxyflurane anaesthesia.
Ethylene glycol poisoning.

The management of calcium oxalate stones due to hyperoxaluria is disappointing. Various drugs such as pyridoxine, cholestyramine and medium-chain triglycerides have been tried but with little effect. Dietary reduction of oxalate-rich foods such as spinach, asparagus, rhubarb and greens should be advised. High fluid intake to reduce the urinary oxalate concentration must be maintained.

**Xanthinuria.** Xanthine stones may form in patients with xanthinuria. This is a rare autosomal recessive condition in which there is a deficiency in the activity of xanthine oxidase which results in elevated plasma xanthine concentration.

Xanthine stones are:
1. Rare, even in patients with xanthinuria.
2. Brown or yellow/brown in colour.
3. Pure xanthine in two-thirds of cases and mixed with uric acid, calcium oxalate or calcium phosphate in the remainder.
4. Not radio-opaque, unless of mixed type, and therefore difficult to detect radiologically.
5. Difficult to diagnose unless suspected and submitted to detailed chemical analysis.

Management is by:
1. High fluid intake.
2. Maintenance of an alkaline urine.
3. Surgical removal if causing pain or obstruction.
4. Careful follow-up.


## HYPERCALCIURIA

The normal urinary excretion of calcium is less than 250 mg daily in females and less than 300 mg daily in males. In the normal person the amount excreted in the urine is equal to the intestinal absorption as a balanced state exists. The intestinal absorption of calcium is only partly related to intake and a considerable increase in oral intake is required to cause a significant rise in urinary excretion.

Hypercalciuria can be caused by:
1. Increased renal loss by abnormal tubular reabsorption; renal tubular acidosis.
2. Increased intestinal absorption; as in vitamin D intoxication and sarcoidosis.
3. Endocrine disease; hyperparathyroidism, Cushing's disease and hyperthyroidism.
4. Bone disease; prolonged immobilization, Paget's disease, carcinomatosis and multiple myeloma.
5. Idiopathic hypercalciuria; characterized by increased calcium excretion, normal plasma calcium and low plasma phosphorus. It is thought to be due to either increased intestinal absorption or a failure of the renal tubule to reabsorb calcium normally.

The management of hypercalciuria is:
1. To determine if there is secondary cause and to treat accordingly.
2. In idiopathic cases to reduce the dietary intake of calcium and maintain a high fluid intake. Thiazide diuretics lower the urinary calcium but the mechanism is not known. Sodium cellulose phosphate which binds calcium in the gut reduces the amount available for absorption.

# Chapter 13

# CONGENITAL AND INHERITED CONDITIONS

Introduction – Cystic renal disease – Inherited glomerular diseases – Inherited tubular disorders

## INTRODUCTION

The classification of inherited diseases of the kidney is difficult as a wide variety of familial conditions affecting the kidney have been described. Many of these conditions are rare and appear to affect only single families. Others are well recognized and the more common will be described in this chapter. Two major problems arise. First, many inherited conditions can also arise as secondary disorders, e.g. renal tubular acidosis may be inherited but can also arise from vitamin D intoxication. Secondly, several systemic conditions can exhibit renal involvement, e.g. oxalosis, familial Mediterranean fever and sickle-cell disease. These are not truly inherited renal diseases but inherited conditions with multisystem involvement.

In this chapter it is convenient to consider: (1) the various forms of cystic disease, (2) inherited glomerular diseases and (3) inherited tubular disorders.

## CYSTIC RENAL DISEASE

**Classification.** The classification of cystic disease of the kidney is difficult; although there are well-recognized clinical syndromes there is also a wide variety of rare forms described in the literature. A satisfactory working classification is:

1. Solitary or simple cysts
2. Polycystic renal disease
   A. Adult type
   B. Infantile type
      Congenital hepatic fibrosis
3. Medullary cystic disease
   A. Medullary sponge kidney
   B. Medullary cystic disease
      Familial juvenile nephronopthisis
      Retinal-renal dysplasia

**Solitary or Simple Cysts.** Simple cysts are common and probably occur in as many as 50 per cent of persons aged over 50 years. Occasionally the simple cysts may be multiple and bilateral.

Frequently these cysts are found as an incidental finding at clinical examination or during pyelography. They are rarely responsible for symptoms although haemorrhage or infection may occur.

Most such cysts are cortical in site and often bulge through the renal capsule. Carcinoma may develop in a simple cyst. The appearances in pyelography may be difficult to interpret and tomography, ultrasound and arteriography may be necessary to differentiate the simple cyst from a carcinoma.

The management is to leave alone unless a carcinoma is suspected. Renal function is not impaired and prognosis is excellent.

**Polycystic Renal Disease.** There are two main types of polycystic disease, an adult type and infantile type.

A. ADULT TYPE. Adult type polycystic renal disease is a relatively common familial condition characterized by the presence of multiple cysts of variable size producing symmetrical enlargement of the kidneys and most commonly becoming clinically apparent in middle age.

*Pathogenesis.* Uncertain, but is due either to:
1. Failure of union of branches of the ureteric bud with the metanephrogenic cap, or
2. Failure of involution and subsequent cyst formation by the first generation of nephrons to differentiate in the metanephros.

*Genetics.* Inherited as a simple autosomal dominant with a high penetrance and a somewhat variable expressivity. It does not occur in the same families as the infantile form.

*Pathology.* The kidneys are almost invariably symmetrically enlarged and may weigh up to 2 kg. Unilateral cases have been rarely reported. The cysts are of variable size up to 5 cm in diameter and contain fluid which may be clear or bloodstained. The cysts are lined by a flattened single layer of epithelium which may resemble the epithelium of proximal tubule, distal tubule or collecting ducts.

*Clinical Presentation.* Most become clinically apparent after the age of 40 years but may present at any age from 8 to 80 years. The modes of presentation are:
1. Haematuria, which may occur after minor trauma and may even produce clot colic.
2. Urinary tract infection.
3. A sensation of heaviness in the loins or the patient noticing abdominal discomfort and distension.
4. Hypertension.
5. Haemorrhage into a cyst with subsequent loin pain.
6. An unexpected finding during a clinical examination.
7. During investigation because of a strong family history.
8. Chronic renal failure.

*Clinical Findings.* By the time symptoms develop the kidneys are usually palpable.

1. The kidneys are symmetrically enlarged and the surface feels irregular.
2. Hypertension is present in approximately 30 per cent of patients at presentation but increases in incidence as renal failure progresses.
3. Renal function may be impaired but the associated anaemia and osteodystrophy may be milder than in patients with other conditions producing a similar reduction in function.
4. Urinary tract infection common.
5. The i.v.p. reveals a characteristic stretching and distortion of the calyces.
6. Ultrasound can confirm the diagnosis.
7. Splenomegaly may be present.
8. There is frequently a family history of kidney disease.
9. The natural history is of a slow but steady decline of renal function.

*Management.* This falls into three categories:
1. From the diagnosis to the onset of terminal renal failure the important points are:
    *a.* Control of hypertension.
    *b.* Control of any urinary tract infection; this may require suppressive antibiotics as it is frequently difficult to eradicate infection from cysts. Antibiotics known to affect renal function, such as tetracyclines, must be avoided.
    *c.* Severe or recurrent haemorrhage is an indication for cystoscopy and angiography.
    *d.* Remember carcinoma may develop in a cyst.
2. The management of terminal renal failure:
    *a.* By the use of dietary restriction of protein, and sodium if hypertension is present.
    *b.* An unhurried assessment as to suitability for haemodialysis.
    *c.* Avoidance of peritoneal dialysis.
    *d.* If suitable for haemodialysis the formation of a fistula once the serum creatinine exceeds 600 $\mu$mol/l with subsequent establishment on dialysis when symptomatic and thus the avoidance of long periods of dietary restrictions.
    *e.* Transplantation; this may require pre-transplant nephrectomy if the kidneys are excessively large.
3. Counselling and screening of relatives:
    *a.* Most patients request genetic counselling. In view of the very variable progression of the condition this is difficult but potential parents should be informed of the 50 per cent chance of any child becoming affected.

*b.* The most effective method of screening of relatives is to monitor blood pressure and examine the kidneys by ultrasound.

*Prognosis.* This is very variable.

1. The younger the patient becomes symptomatic the poorer the prognosis.
2. Once there is evidence of decline in renal function terminal renal failure is commonly reached within 3 years.
3. The presence of hypertension or repeated urinary tract infections infers a poorer prognosis.
4. Rarely carcinoma develops in a cyst, the frequency of which is not known.
5. The causes of death are approximately: uraemia 50 per cent; myocardial infarction 10 per cent; cerebral haemorrhage 10 per cent; congestive cardiac failure 10 per cent and unrelated causes 20 per cent.

*Associated Abnormalities*

1. Approximately 30 per cent have hepatic cysts but these produce no functional impairment.
2. Cysts in the pancreas and/or spleen.
3. Some 15 per cent of patients have aneurysms of the cerebral arteries and subarachnoid haemorrhage is a cause of death in approximately 10 per cent of patients.

B. INFANTILE TYPE. Infantile type polycystic renal disease is a rare condition in which there is gross bilateral cystic enlargement of both kidneys which may be so severe as to interfere with delivery. It is probably inherited as autosomal recessive which is thus manifest only in homozygotes.

The kidneys are composed of multiple fusiform or cylindrical cysts which appear to be radially orientated and frequently obscure the corticomedullary junction. The pathogenesis is unknown. There are probably several distinct varieties. In some cases there is cystic proliferation of the bile ducts in the liver and occasionally cysts in the lung and pancreas.

The clinical presentation is the obvious renal enlargement usually present at birth. The majority of patients die from renal failure in the perinatal period although some may live for several years.

Congenital hepatic fibrosis is a form of infantile polycystic disease in which there is renal cystic disease and portal fibrosis leading to portal hypertension. The majority of patients present with symptoms of portal hypertension in their second decade. The first symptom is frequently sudden massive upper gastrointestinal bleeding. Ascites, splenomegaly and collateral venous circulations are features. Hepatic and renal function are usually good but death occurs from progressive portal hypertension.

**Medullary Cystic Disease.** The two major conditions in which cysts are present predominantly in the medulla are medullary sponge kidney and medullary cystic disease.

A. MEDULLARY SPONGE KIDNEY. An uncommon condition characterized by the presence of multiple small cysts in some or all of the pyramids of the kidney. The cysts frequently contain small calculi.

*Pathogenesis.* Unknown.

*Genetics.* Familial but not hereditary. It is twice as common in males as females.

*Pathology.* Multiple cystic dilatation of papillary collecting ducts. The cysts frequently contain small calculi and debris. Cysts are not present in the cortex.

*Clinical Presentation.* Frequently asymptomatic but when symptoms occur it is usually after the fourth decade and may present as:
   1. Renal colic due to the spontaneous passage of small calculi.
   2. Dysuria due to urinary tract infection.
   3. Haematuria.
   4. Bilateral loin pain.

*Clinical Findings.*
   1. Kidneys may be modestly enlarged, normal or small depending upon the extent of secondary pyelonephritis.
   2. Glomerular filtration is usually normal.
   3. Urinary concentrating ability is frequently impaired.
   4. Excretion of acid impaired.
   5. Hypercalciuria may occur.
   6. I.v.p. shows contrast media in the cysts in the medulla and the pyramids may be enlarged. On plain X-ray there may be multiple clusters of calculi in calyceal pyramids.

*Management.* There is no curative treatment.
   1. Monitor and treat any infection.
   2. High fluid intake.
   3. Prevention of renal calculi.

*Prognosis.* Generally good depending on the extent of pyelonephritis and the damage from calculi.

B. MEDULLARY CYSTIC DISEASE. A rare, probably familial condition, in which there are multiple cysts mainly in the medulla and particularly at the corticomedullary junction. Small cysts may also appear in the cortex.

It is probably a heterogeneous group of familial nephropathies which include familial juvenile nephronopthisis and retinal-renal dysplasia.

*Clinical Presentation.* Usually becomes manifest in adolescents and young adults:
   1. Anaemia.

2. Polyuria.
3. Chronic renal failure.
4. 'Salt-losing nephropathy'.

*Clinical Findings*
1. Small kidneys.
2. Uraemia.
3. Inability to concentrate urine.
4. Metabolic acidosis.

*Management*
1. Symptomatic.
2. High fluid intake; diarrhoea and vomiting may precipitate reversible deterioration in renal function and frequently requires intravenous fluid replacement.
3. Sodium supplements.
4. Bicarbonate supplements.
5. Consideration for dialysis and transplantation as and when necessary.

*Prognosis.* Poor with eventual deterioration of renal function to terminal renal failure.

## INHERITED GLOMERULAR DISEASES

**Introduction.** Inherited glomerular diseases are not common. There is increasing evidence that certain forms of glomerulonephritis have HLA associations and so the mode of inheritance of these conditions may with time become more clear. The most commonly recognized inherited glomerular condition is Alport's syndrome.

**Alport's Syndrome.** A syndrome characterized by a hereditary glomerulonephritis, perceptive nerve deafness and, in some cases, eye abnormalities (spherophakia, cataracts, lenticonus). The sex incidence is probably equal but males are more severely affected and carry a much poorer prognosis. It is uncommon for females to be symptomatic before the age of 40 while most males have entered terminal renal failure by the age of 30. It is inherited as autosomal dominant with variable penetrance and expressivity.

Clinical presentation:
1. Haematuria: the most common presentation and may occur in association with upper respiratory tract infection or spontaneously.
2. Deafness.
3. Hypertension.
4. Chronic renal failure.

The clinical findings depend to a large extent on the age and sex of the patient. The deafness is of a perceptive type with initially particular loss of the high tone frequencies. Vestibular branch function is normal. Proteinuria is usually mild and glycosuria has been reported in a significant number of patients. The natural history in male patients is of progressive renal failure while in the females this is uncommon and when present occurs at a much older age.

The renal lesion is a proliferative glomerulonephritis which in some cases has a focal accentuation. On electron microscopy the basement membrane shows focal or diffuse splitting in which lucent areas containing small moderately dense granulations appear to separate darker staining layers of membrane. In the interstitium there are patchy areas of tubular loss, inflammatory cell infiltrate and interstitial fibrosis.

The management is by control of hypertension and that of chronic renal failure. The prognosis in males is poor whilst in females it is much better.

**Fabry's Disease (Angiokeratoma Corporis Diffusum Universale).** A rare condition involving the skin, kidneys, heart and CNS. The skin lesions consist of small dark red papules which have some hyperkeratosis. These lesions tend to occur on the trunk, particularly peri-umbilical. There is an X-linked error of glycosphingolipid metabolism with an accumulation of ceramide trihexoside in cells. The skin manifestations are more marked in males than females.

The disease usually becomes manifest before puberty and renal failure is the most common cause of death. The glomeruli show a fine foamy vacuolation of the epithelial cells and later hyalinization. There is no known therapy but it has been reported that transplantation results in considerable improvement in symptoms with a return to normal of plasma and urine ceramide trihexoside and this may be due to correction of the inborn error of metabolism by enzymes in the transplanted kidney.

**Congenital Nephrotic Syndrome.** A rare familial condition which is autosomal recessive with an increased incidence in Finland. Affected children are usually born pre-term, have a low birth weight and an abnormally large placenta. Proteinuria and oedema may be present at birth but usually become manifest within the first 2 months of life. Pathologically the kidneys may be normal or increased in size, in the glomeruli there may be patchy thickening of the capillary wall and basement membrane while the proximal tubules show marked cystic dilatation.

The condition is fatal and there is no response to steroid therapy. Death usually occurs in the first 2 years with only 25 per cent of patients surviving beyond the first year. The cause of death is usually infection but may be any complication of severe nephrotic syndrome.

**Nail-patella Syndrome (Hereditary Osteo-onychodysplasia).** A rare autosomal dominant condition in which there is hypoplasia or absence of the patellae, subluxation of the radial heads at the elbow and dysplasia of the finger nails associated with glomerulonephritis. The renal lesion is of a patchy thickening of glomerular basement membrane leading eventually to complete sclerosis. There may also be marked thickening of the tubular basement membrane. The prognosis is variable but a significant number progress to uraemia.

## INHERITED TUBULAR DISORDERS

**Introduction.** Inherited renal tubular disorders may affect virtually any function of the tubule. The majority of syndromes are rare and so only the more common forms will be described. The tubular defect may be single or multiple and involve (1) either abnormal excretion or reabsorption of a substance or group of substances, or (2) the failure of the nephron to respond to circulating hormones, e.g. nephrogenic diabetes insipidus.

### Proximal Tubule

CYSTINURIA. A syndrome characterized by a disturbance in the proximal tubular handling of the amino acids cystine, ornithine, arginine and lysine (COAL). Similar transport defects occur in the intestinal mucosa.

Clinically, these patients present with renal calculi. Cystine stones account for approximately 1 per cent of all calculi but are of importance as the majority of such patients present before the age of 30 and frequently have bilateral recurrent stones. Large amounts of the amino acids (up to 4 g daily) are excreted in the urine and microscopy may show the presence of typical hexagonal crystals. The calculi are radio-opaque.

Two types of cystinuria are recognized. The first and most common is *recessive cystinuria* where only those patients homozygous for the defect excrete abnormal amounts of COAL. The second is *incompletely recessive* where heterozygous patients excrete intermediate amounts and the remaining members of the families excrete normal amino acids.

The management of the homozygous patients who are stone formers is:

1. Maintain a high urine flow rate, at least 3 l daily. One should aim to keep a high flow rate at night.
2. Maintain an alkaline urine by the administration of bicarbonate.
3. Penicillamine has been used but it may be associated with unpleasant side effects.

HARTNUP DISEASE. A very rare autosomal recessive condition presenting clinically with photosensitivity, skin rash resembling pellagra and attacks of cerebellar ataxia. Attacks occur in childhood and tend to become less frequent with age.

The amino acid transport defects involve alanine, glutamine, asparagine, histidine, serine, threonine, phenylalanine, tyrosine and tryptophan. There is an intestinal abnormality in the transport

of tryptophan and this results in an increased breakdown of tryptophan in the gut with consequent increased indol formation. As a
result there is increased excretion of indols in the urine. Apart
from the tubular amino acid transport abnormality there are no
other tubular transport defects.

CYSTINOSIS (LIGNAC–FANCONI SYNDROME). A rare autosomal
recessive condition in which there is deposition of cystine in many
organs associated with defective proximal tubular transport
mechanism.

The condition is usually manifest in childhood and two types
are recognized:

1. An acute form which is usually recognized by 6 months and
   presents as failure to thrive, polyuria and polydipsia. The
   prognosis is extremely poor and death, usually from infection, is frequent before the end of the first decade.
2. A chronic form which usually presents as D-resistant rickets
   and death is usually from chronic renal failure in adolescence.

In both forms there are multiple proximal tubular transport
defects leading to: glycosuria; generalized amino aciduria; hyperphosphaturia; acidosis (due to renal bicarbonate wasting); hypokalaemia; tubular proteinuria; hypo-uricaemia; rickets (due to
vitamin D deficiency).

In the chronic form the amino aciduria and glycosuria are less
than in the acute form.

Cystine deposits are found in the reticulo-endothelial system,
leucocytes, fibroblasts, the kidney and the cornea of the eye. The
kidney shows sclerotic glomeruli and hexagonal crystals of cystine
can be detected in cells by electron microscopy. There is tubular
atrophy and the proximal tubule may show a narrow segment which
has been termed the 'swan-neck deformity'.

The prognosis in both acute and chronic forms is poor and
treatment symptomatic.

A similar condition occurs in adults rarely as a familial disease
and more commonly as an acquired condition (*see* Chapter 14,
p. 158). It usually presents as muscle weakness and osteomalacia
and is associated with the deposition of cystine.

RENAL GLYCOSURIA. A relatively common defect in proximal
tubular handling of glucose and occurs in approximately 2 per cent
of the population. Glycosuria is the only abnormality and is due to
decrease in the maximum tubular glucose reabsorption. It is differentiated from diabetes mellitus by finding:

1. Glycosuria without hyperglycaemia.
2. Normal fasting blood glucose.
3. Normal or flat glucose tolerance test.

VITAMIN D-RESISTANT RICKETS. This unusual condition is a rare

X-linked dominant condition although sporadic cases have an autosomal dominant inheritance. It is characterized by: hypophosphataemia; rickets or osteomalacia not responsive to physiological amounts of vitamin D; abnormal vitamin D metabolism associated with diminished intestinal absorption of calcium and phosphate; increased renal phosphate clearance.

The clinical presentation is usually as rickets in childhood. It is not associated with any other renal tubular abnormalities. Treatment is with large doses of vitamin D or its analogues and should be started early to prevent permanent skeletal deformity.

RENAL TUBULAR ACIDOSIS (TYPE 2). As a primary disease this is rare (secondary form, *see* p. 156). It is due to impairment of the proximal tubular sodium-hydrogen exchange with a consequent 'leak' of bicarbonate so that an inappropriate amount of bicarbonate appears in the urine for a given plasma concentration.

The clinical presentation is in infancy with failure to thrive, repeated episodes of vomiting and a hyperchloraemic acidosis in the presence of an alkaline or very slightly acid urine. Unlike distal tubular acidosis bone disease and nephrocalcinosis are rare. The management is to provide large amounts of alkali as bicarbonate 6–10 mmol/kg/day, half as the sodium salt and half as potassium salt. The prognosis is good and the biochemical disturbances may become less in later life and it may be possible to stop therapy.

**Distal Tubule**

FAMILIAL NEPHROGENIC DIABETES INSIPIDUS. A rare inherited condition in which the distal tubule and collecting duct are unresponsive to ADH. The affected infants have intense polyuria and severe dehydration may result. Early diagnosis is essential as permanent mental deficiency may result from the prolonged severe dehydration.

The defect is in the epithelial cells where there is probably a deficiency in cyclic AMP.

Autosomal dominant and sex-linked inheritance patterns have been described.

RENAL TUBULAR ACIDOSIS (TYPE 1). The primary form of this disease usually presents in the first 18 months of life (secondary form, *see* p. 154). The clinical features are failure to thrive, polyuria, dehydration and constipation. Some cases are detected following investigation of growth failure. The pathophysiology is a failure of distal tubular hydrogen ion secretion either because the distal tubular cells fail to generate $H^+$ ions or there is a failure in the excretion of $H^+$ ions into the tubular lumen.

In patients with this form of renal tubular acidosis there is invariably nephrocalcinosis and renal stones, rickets/osteomalacia

*Table* 13.1. Inheritance of renal diseases

| | |
|---|---|
| *Cystic Diseases* | |
|     Adult polycystic | AD |
|     Infantile polycystic | AR |
| *Glomerular Diseases* | |
|     Alport's syndrome | AD |
|     Fabry's disease | XL |
|     Congenital nephrotic syndrome | AR |
|     Nail-patella syndrome | AD |
| *Tubular Disorders* | |
|     Proximal Tubule | |
|       Cystinuria | AR |
|       Hartnup disease | AR |
|       Cystinosis | AR |
|       Renal glycosuria | AD |
|       Renal tubular acidosis (Type 2) | AD |
|       Vitamin D-resistant rickets | XL |
|     Distal Tubule | |
|       Renal tubular acidosis (Type 1) | AD |
|       Familial nephrogenic diabetes insipidus | XL |

AD, Autosomal dominant.
AR, Autosomal recessive.
XL, X-linked.

and muscle weakness are common. Diagnosis is by finding a failure to acidify the urine in the presence of a systemic acidosis or failure to drop the urine pH below 5·4 after an ammonium chloride load. Treatment is with bicarbonate 1–3 mmol/kg/day, potassium supplements and vitamin D if bony problems are severe and not responding to correction of the acidosis. In acute situations considerable potassium supplements may be required. Urinary tract infection needs to be treated promptly. Prognosis is good unless there has been significant destruction of renal tissue from nephrocalcinosis or the development of hypertension or chronic urinary tract infection.

# Chapter 14

# RENAL TUBULAR DISEASE AND MISCELLANEOUS CONDITIONS

Renal tubular acidosis – Interstitial nephritis – Balkan nephropathy – Fanconi syndrome – Metal toxicity – Disorders of urinary concentration – Radiation nephritis – The kidney in liver disease – The kidney in pregnancy – Retroperitoneal fibrosis – Sickle-cell disease – Bartter's syndrome – Segmental hypoplasia (Ask–Upmark kidney) – Tumours

## RENAL TUBULAR ACIDOSIS

Metabolic acidosis develops in renal disease due to: (1) a reduction in renal mass producing an inability to excrete hydrogen ions, or (2) an impairment in either proximal or distal tubular function resulting in failure to maintain the normal plasma bicarbonate concentration. In conditions where the glomerular filtration falls below 20 ml/min there is impairment in $H^+$ secretion resulting in metabolic acidosis as part of the syndrome of uraemia. In renal tubular disease, however, there is frequently little or no reduction in renal function, and the metabolic acidosis which develops is known as renal tubular acidosis (RTA). The major abnormality may occur in the distal tubule producing classic or Type 1 RTA or in the proximal tubule producing Type 2 RTA.

**Distal Renal Tubular Acidosis (Classic, Type 1).** In the distal form there is failure of urinary acidification, despite severe systemic acidosis, due to either failure of the distal tubular cells to generate $H^+$ or failure of the distal tubule to excrete $H^+$. Two forms of this condition have been described, the first where there is persistent hyperchloraemic acidosis known as *complete* and the second, *incomplete*, where there are normal acid-base parameters but an inability to excrete an acid load.

The clinical presentation is usually with anorexia, fatigue, muscle weakness, osteomalacia, nephrocalcinosis and nephrolithiasis.

Associated with the metabolic acidosis there may be:
1. Renal sodium wasting due to diminished hydrogen–sodium exchange in the distal tubule.
2. Potassium depletion consequent on stimulation of the renin–angiotensin–aldosterone system by volume depletion from sodium wasting.
3. Hypercalciuria.
4. Increased clearance of phosphate.
5. Recurrent stone formation from the increased urinary calcium and phosphate excretion.
6. Nephrocalcinosis (as 5).
7. Hypocalcaemia from interference with vitamin D metabolism. The

1α hydroxylation by the kidney is inhibited by the acidosis. Hypo-calcaemia may also be aggravated by the hypercalciuria.

8. Osteomalacia, or rickets from abnormal vitamin D metabolism (as 7).

There are many clinical disorders which can cause Type 1 RTA:

Primary (Chapter 13, p. 152)

Secondary

    Dysproteinaemias
        Hyperglobulinaemia
        Cryoglobulinaemia
        Amyloidosis
    Disordered calcium metabolism
        Vitamin D intoxication
        Hyperparathyroidism
        Idiopathic hypercalciuria
    Immunologically mediated diseases
        Chronic active hepatitis
        Primary biliary cirrhosis
        Sjögren's syndrome
        Systemic lupus erythematosus
    Drug induced
        Lithium
        Amphotericin B
    Renal diseases
        Pyelonephritis
        Medullary sponge kidney
        Hydronephrosis
        Transplantation
    Miscellaneous
        Sickle-cell disease
        Wilson's disease

Management is by, where possible, determining the underlying cause of the RTA. Treatment must then be directed to the primary pathology. The renal tubular acidosis is treated by:

1. Bicarbonate supplements, in the region of 2 mmol/kg body weight/day. The exact dose can only be determined by trial but the aim should be to keep the plasma bicarbonate in excess of 18 mmol/l.

2. Calcium and vitamin D may be required if bicarbonate replacement and correction of the acidosis does not relieve the bone pain and hypercalciuria.

3. Potassium supplements may be required in the initial treatment as there can be profound potassium depletion.

The prognosis is related to the underlying cause of the RTA. Correction of the acidosis is usually associated with a return to normal calcium and phosphate metabolism and thus a diminution of stone formation.

**Proximal Renal Tubular Acidosis (Type 2).** This usually occurs as part of a complex of proximal tubular disorders consisting of glycosuria, aminoaciduria, phosphaturia and uricosuria. There is impairment of proximal tubular sodium—hydrogen exchange decreasing bicarbonate resorption. This results in bicarbonate wasting and a reduction in the plasma bicarbonate. The filtered load of bicarbonate falls and when this matches the diminished proximal tubular activity a new steady state is achieved. Bicarbonate wasting then ceases and this allows for acidification of the urine and thus patients are able to excrete their daily acid load.

The RTA is associated with:

1. Hyperchloraemia; due to sodium wasting there is stimulation of the renin—angiotensin—aldosterone system with retention of sodium chloride.
2. Potassium depletion, due to secondary aldosteronism.
3. Hypocalcaemia, but unlike distal RTA there is seldom bone disease or nephrocalcinosis.

Many clinical syndromes are associated with proximal RTA:

Primary (Chapter 13, p. 152)

Secondary

    Disorders of amino acid metabolism
        Cystinosis
        Tyrosinosis
    Heavy metal toxicity
        Cadmium
        Lead
        Copper
        Mercury
    Drug induced
        Tetracycline
        Carbonic anhydrase inhibitors
        6-Mercaptopurine
    Renal diseases
        Nephrotic syndrome
        Amyloidosis
        Transplantation
    Miscellaneous
        Multiple myeloma
        Sjögren's syndrome
        Hyperparathyroidism
        Vitamin D toxicity

Management is aimed at the underlying cause and at relief of the acidosis.

1. In adults if the plasma bicarbonate is greater than 18 mmol/l then bicarbonate supplements are not required.
2. If plasma bicarbonate below 18 mmol/l then sodium bicarbonate

in an appropriate dose, in the range 2–10 mmol/kg body weight/day.

3. In children bicarbonate supplements are usually required and there may also be a need for vitamin D and calcium supplements.

## INTERSTITIAL NEPHRITIS

The term 'interstitial nephritis' is used to describe a number of conditions where the main reaction appears to be in the interstitium and where there is frequently tubular damage with little or no glomerular abnormality.

*Acute interstitial nephritis* frequently presents as acute renal failure and is commonly due to a drug reaction. There is frequently an accompanying fever, skin rash and eosinophilia. Haematuria is common but proteinuria is seldom greater than 2 g daily. The drugs implicated have included:

| | |
|---|---|
| Methicillin | Phenindione |
| Sulphonamides | Penicillin |
| Rifampicin | Ampicillin |
| Diphenylhydantoin | Analgesics |
| Metals | Diuretics |

On renal biopsy there is considerable interstitial oedema and infiltration with lymphocytes, plasma cells, polymorphs and eosinophils. The tubules may show a variety of changes from normal to necrosis. On withdrawal of the drug the renal lesions usually resolve.

Management is by withdrawing the drug or precipitating agent providing this is known. If the lesion is severe enough to produce acute renal failure this should be managed along conventional lines (Chapter 7).

*Chronic interstitial nephritis* frequently presents with symptoms of polyuria, nocturia, polydypsia, anaemia and hypertension. There may be a surprising lack of symptoms even in the presence of severely impaired renal function. On investigation, however, there is frequently increased urine volume, renal tubular acidosis, potassium depletion and a sodium-losing state. The renal biopsy reveals interstitial oedema and infiltration with lymphocytes and plasma cells; in longstanding cases there may be considerable tubular atrophy and fibrosis. Glomeruli may have varying degrees of hyalinization. There are many causes including:

Drug induced
    Analgesic abuse
    Heavy metal exposure
Metabolic disease
    Cystinosis
    Gout
    Diabetes mellitus
Immunological
    Transplant rejection
    SLE

      Rapidly progressive glomerulonephritis
      Sjögren's syndrome
  Infections
      Pyelonephritis
      Leptospirosis
  Miscellaneous
      Sickle-cell disease
      Balkan nephropathy
      Irradiation

Management is by careful control of fluid and electrolyte balance. There may be a need for sodium, potassium and bicarbonate supplements. Control of hypertension and uraemia is by standard regimens.

## BALKAN NEPHROPATHY

This is a particular form of interstitial nephritis which occurs within a fairly well circumscribed area in Romania, Bulgaria and Yugoslavia. It is most common in agricultural areas and there is a considerable variation in the incidence from village to village. In some communities the incidence is as great as 60 per cent. Males and females are equally affected with a peak age incidence between 30 and 40 years.

The clinical presentation is insidious with bilateral loin pain, anorexia and weakness. There is frequently an unusual yellow skin pigmentation particularly of the palms of the hands. Hypertension is uncommon. Renal failure is slowly progressive and death usually occurs some five years after initial presentation.

The distal tubule appears to the initially affected with subsequent involvement of the whole nephron. There is marked tubular loss with interstitial fibrosis and glomerular hyalinization. There is frequently malignant tumours of the urinary tract.

The management is directed mainly at the underlying renal failure. There is no specific therapy.

## FANCONI SYNDROME

The Fanconi syndrome is characterized by: osteomalacia; glycosuria; generalized aminoaciduria; hypokalaemia; acidosis; hyperphosphaturia.

It may occur as a familial condition (*see* Chapter 13, p. 151) in both adults and children. It occurs more commonly in adults as an acquired disease and it usually presents as muscle weakness and osteomalacia.

It is due to disturbance of the normal proximal tubular transport mechanisms and this leads to an excessive urinary loss of glucose, amino acids, potassium, bicarbonate and phosphate. It may be acquired in a wide variety of clinical situations:

  Immunological diseases
      Myeloma

    Amyloidosis
    Light chain disease
    Systemic lupus erythematosus
    Sjögren's syndrome
    Interstitial nephritis with anti-GBM antibody
    Connective tissue diseases
    Renal transplantation
Drugs
    Outdated tetracycline
    6-Mercaptopurine
Metals
    Cadmium
    Lead
    Mercury
Balkan nephropathy
Wilson's disease
The management of acquired Fanconi syndrome:

1. Control of the underlying pathology.
2. Correction of hypokalaemia with oral potassium supplements.
3. Correction of the metabolic acidosis with sodium bicarbonate supplements.
4. Control of the osteomalacia with either vitamin D or one of the newer synthetic analogues.

## METAL TOXICITY

A number of metals can give rise to renal damage. Commonly this is tubular, producing glycosuria, aminoaciduria and tubular proteinuria but in some instances (gold and possibly mercury) there may also be glomerular lesions.

**Lead.** Usually the systemic manifestations of intestinal colic, peripheral neuropathy, anaemia and encephalopathy are more apparent than the nephropathy. In patients with renal involvement there is hypertension, slowly progressive renal failure and gouty symptoms from hyperuricaemia. The lead is absorbed by inhalation from the burning of lead paint or lead batteries or by gut absorption from lead-contaminated water. The renal lesion is mainly tubular, leading to glycosuria, aminoaciduria and protein-uria. The proximal tubular cells show characteristic eosinophilic intranuclear inclusion bodies containing a lead-protein complex.

Management is to (*a*) cease exposure to lead, (*b*) increase excretion by chelation, (*c*) control hypertension, symptoms of gout, and uraemia by standard means.

**Gold.** The clinical manifestations of gold toxicity are cutaneous hyper-sensitivity, marrow suppression and the nephrotic syndrome. Proteinuria occurs in some 5 per cent of patients receiving therapeutic gold. In addition there may be microscopic haematuria and uraemia may develop. The renal lesion is an irregular thickening of the glomerular basement membrane but in some patients there may be only minimal changes. Management is by withdrawal of gold therapy and symptomatic treatment of the oedema and renal failure.

**Cadmium.** Toxicity is mainly associated with the manufacture of batteries and contamination of water supplies. The clinical presentation is with painful osteomalacia, respiratory symptoms, loss of smell, nephrolithiasis, emphysema and impaired renal function. The renal damage is predominantly to the proximal tubule and is associated with glycosuria, aminoaciduria, renal tubular acidosis and low molecular weight proteinuria. $\beta_2$-microglobulin excretion is greatly increased. Interstitial fibrosis occurs. Management is removal of the source and supportive treatment for the painful osteomalacia, renal tubular acidosis and nephrolithiasis.

**Beryllium.** Toxicity is usually due to exposure to fumes during fluorescent light manufacture. The renal lesion is described as a chronic granulomatous interstitial nephritis.

**Mercury.** Acute toxicity causes acute renal failure due to necrosis of proximal tubular cells. Chronic exposure results in impaired renal function and in the kidney there are minor glomerular changes associated with a flattening of the proximal tubular epithelium.

**Arsenic and Bismuth.** In acute poisoning changes similar to that seen in mercury toxicity are found.

**Copper.** In Wilson's disease copper may accumulate in the proximal tubular cells producing aminoaciduria.


## DISORDERS OF URINARY CONCENTRATION

Inability to concentrate urine can be due to a lack of antidiuretic hormone (ADH) or an inability of the kidney to respond to circulating ADH.

A lack of ADH (diabetes insipidus) results from damage to the hypothalamic–pituitary axis producing a permanent or transient reduction in ADH secretion.

Trauma

Tumours (primary or secondary)

Pituitary irradiation

Inflammatory lesions

Granulomatous lesions

An inability of the kidney to respond to ADH (nephrogenic diabetes insipidus) produces a large volume of dilute urine and may be caused by:

Inability of loop of Henle to form an adequate medullary solute gradient.

Hypokalaemia

    Hypercalcaemia
    Osmotic diuresis (uraemia)
    Malnutrition
Medullary disease with structural damage to the loops of Henle.
    Analgesic nephropathy
    Hydronephrosis
    Chronic pyelonephritis
    Nephrocalcinosis
    Medullary cystic disease
    Sickle-cell disease
'Washout' of medullary solute gradient.
    Acute tubular necrosis
    Urinary obstruction
    Sustained excessive water drinking
Drug induced.
    Outdated tetracycline
    Demethylchlortetracycline
    Amphotericin

The diagnosis of defects of urinary concentration involves a careful history and clinical examination followed by tests to determine whether the kidney can or cannot respond to ADH. Overnight concentration tests with and without ADH are performed (*see* Chapter 3).

The treatment has improved with the introduction of synthetic analogues of ADH. Other drugs are also of value:

1. Lysine-vasopressin; administered by nasal spray, short lasting effect is inconvenient.
2. Desmopressin (DDAVP, Desamino-D-Arginine Vasopressin); twice daily nasal administration usually produces effective control.
3. Chlorpropamide; of value in diabetes insipidus but not in the nephrogenic form. It acts by potentiating the effect of ADH on the collecting duct and possibly also by promoting its central release.
4. Clofibrate; action probably by facilitating release of ADH.
5. Diuretics; paradoxically reduce urine volume in diabetes insipidus probably by their ability to interfere with sodium transport in the ascending limb of the loop of Henle and thus preventing dilute urine from passing on to the distal part of the nephron.

## RADIATION NEPHRITIS

Irradiation injury to the kidneys may follow radiotherapy to abdominal organs or lymph nodes. There is a very considerable variation in patient susceptibility to radiation injury. Two clinical syndromes are recognized, acute and chronic radiation nephritis.

Acute radiation nephritis usually occurs 6–12 months after toxic doses, earlier in children. Presentation is with oedema, hypertension, dyspnoea, headaches, anaemia and proteinuria. The hypertension is usually the first sign and this frequently returns to normal as the episode subsides. The proteinuria is *mild* and rarely in excess of 4 g/24 hours. The anaemia is severe, normochromic, normocytic. The prognosis is variable with a 50 per cent mortality in the acute phase. In other patients recovery is associated with an improvement in hypertension and an increase in renal function although proteinuria may continue for years.

Chronic radiation nephritis usually appears several years after radiation. There may have been a preceding acute radiation nephritis or it may appear *de novo* up to 15 years later. Presentation is with fatigue, nocturia, anaemia, hypertension, proteinuria and uraemia. Hypertension is present in 50 per cent of patients and many have a malignant phase. A number of patients will also have evidence of irradiation injury to the gastrointestinal tract and/or pancreas; retroperitoneal fibrosis may also be present. The uraemia is usually slowly progressive. The kidneys from patients with chronic damage are contracted and show sclerosis of glomeruli, tubular loss, fibrinoid necrosis of arterioles and small interlobular arteries and interstitial fibrosis.

Management is by:
1. Control of hypertension. Where there is evidence of unilateral disease or involvement of only part of a kidney removal of the affected tissue may resolve the hypertension.
2. Investigation for possible obstructive uropathy from retroperitoneal fibrosis.
3. The standard management of chronic renal failure (*see* Chapter 8, p. 72).

## THE KIDNEY IN LIVER DISEASE

A variety of liver diseases are associated with renal abnormalities.

**Cirrhosis.** The hepatorenal syndrome is unexplained renal failure occurring in patients with cirrhosis. It is most likely produced by an alteration in renal blood flow due to either a redistribution of the extrarenal circulation or the response to some humoral factor produced or inadequately removed by the diseased liver. In cirrhosis there is also impaired sodium excretion and an inability to excrete a water load. An increase in glomerular mesangium leading to sclerosis is found in a number of patients.

**Hepatitis.** In acute viral hepatitis there may be transient proteinuria and haematuria during the acute phase of the illness. Renal function is normal although there may be mild transient glomerular lesions.

In hepatitis B antigenaemia polyarteritis-like lesions may be found in arterioles while in chronic antigenaemia a membranous glomerulonephritis is described.

Chronic active hepatitis is associated with renal tubular acidosis and this has also been described in cirrhosis and in primary biliary cirrhosis.

**Obstructive Jaundice.** There is a high incidence of acute renal failure and if surgery is contemplated it should be performed under a mannitol diuresis.

**Leptospirosis.** Associated with acute renal failure.

**Cystic Disease.** Patients with adult type polycystic renal disease frequently have liver cysts but these never produce hepatic impairment. Some patients with infantile type polycystic disease have portal fibrosis leading to portal hypertension.


## THE KIDNEY IN PREGNANCY

During pregnancy there are certain changes in renal function and structure.
1. The renal plasma flow increases by approximately 50 per cent during the first trimester and remains elevated until delivery.
2. The glomerular filtration rate also increases by about 50 per cent during the first trimester and likewise remains elevated until delivery.
3. Glycosuria is common due to an increased filtered load from the increased GFR and to a diminution in TmG.
4. Uric acid and histidine excretion are increased.
5. Renin secretion is increased and there is an increase in the aldosterone secretion rate. There is an increase in total body sodium.
6. There is dilatation of the renal tract, particularly the ureters, and this is more marked on the right side. The cause is considered to be pressure from the gravid uterus and the smooth muscle effect of progesterone. After delivery the dilatation regresses over the ensuing six weeks but mild right-sided dilatation may persist for years.


Renal disease in pregnancy has many causes although some are conditions unique to pregnancy. The most common problems are:
Infections
Pre-eclampsia and eclampsia
Glomerulonephritis
Acute renal failure
Chronic renal failure

**Infections** are common in pregnancy, occurring in approximately 5 per cent of women. Asymptomatic bacteriuria is important as about half will progress to pyelonephritis at a later stage in the pregnancy. The reason for the high incidence is the dilatation of the ureter and pelvis with the consequent slowing or urine flow associated with the increased incidence of glycosuria. Infections in pregnancy must be effectively treated otherwise there is an increased chance of permanent renal damage, hypertension and pre-eclampsia.

**Pre-eclampsia and eclampsia** are syndromes which are peculiar to pregnancy. Pre-eclampsia is a syndrome triad consisting of proteinuria, hypertension and oedema. It is more common in primipara and those with pre-existing hypertension, or twin pregnancy. The majority present in the third trimester, 95 per cent occur after the 30th week. The aetiology is unknown but localized intravascular coagulation would appear to be an important pathogenic mechanism.

Clinically there is considerable oedema although the urinary protein seldom exceeds 5 g daily. Hypertension is moderate with a diastolic pressure of up to 110 mmHg. The severity of pre-eclampsia is variable. Patients may progress to a more severe illness with diastolic blood pressures greater than 110 mmHg associated with oliguria, rising plasma creatinine, cerebral and visual disturbances, hyperbilirubinaemia and in some patients pulmonary oedema.

Renal biopsy reveals a mild proliferation of mesangial cells and a marked swelling of the endothelial cells. On electron microscopy there is obvious endotheliosis and in some cases patchy thickening of the basement membrane due to the subendothelial deposition of finely granular or fibrillar material which may be fibrin.

Management is by control of blood pressure and oedema. Pre-eclampsia subsides after delivery.

Eclampsia is where pre-eclampsia progresses to hypertensive encephalopathy with convulsions and coma. This is a medical emergency and urgent delivery should be undertaken. The renal lesion is essentially that of pre-eclampsia but it may be more severe and accompanied by glomerular capillary thromboses and occasionally acute tubular necrosis.

**Glomerulonephritis** arising during pregnancy is difficult to distinguish from pre-eclampsia and if there is doubt renal biopsy should be performed. In the presence of a gravid uterus it is preferable to perform the biopsy with the patient in the sitting position.

Patients with glomerulonephritis who become pregnant have a variable prognosis. The presence of an existing glomerulonephritis is not in itself grounds for recommending termination. Many patients with mild proliferative lesions will progress through their pregnancy with no problems but there is an undoubted increased risk of hypertension becoming apparent or more severe. In patients with a glomerulonephritis causing impaired renal function, serum creatinine in excess of 200 $\mu$mol/l, and hypertension there is an increased risk of (1) deterioration in renal function, (2) increasing severity of hypertension, (3) deterioration in the renal histology, (4) increased fetal loss and (5) increased chance of a low birth weight baby. Patients with mesangiocapillary glomerulonephritis appear to have a poor chance of a successful outcome of pregnancy. All patients with glomerulonephritis who become pregnant require very careful monitoring during pregnancy, parturition and post-partum.

**Acute Renal Failure** arising in pregnancy may be due to: hyperemesis gravidarum; septic abortion; eclampsia; abruptio placentae; postpartum haemorrhage, and, in addition, the many other causes listed in Chapter 7.

Many of these patients develop acute tubular necrosis but there is a high risk of cortical necrosis developing, particularly in abruptio placentae and postpartum haemorrhage. The management of the acute renal failure is along conventional lines (*see* Chapter 7, p. 59) except that peritoneal dialysis is likely to be hazardous due to the gravid uterus and renal biopsy is probably undertaken more frequently to distinguish tubular necrosis from cortical necrosis.

A syndrome of *postpartum acute renal failure* has been described where acute renal failure develops one day to several weeks after delivery. It is frequently accompanied by a 'flu-like illness and a microangiopathic haemolytic anaemia. Hypertension is variable but there is frequently cardiomegaly and cardiac failure. The cause is not known. It is usually irreversible.

**Chronic Renal Failure** is associated with diminished fertility and a high incidence of fetal loss. A serum creatinine in excess of 200 $\mu$mol/l especially in the presence of hypertension significantly increases the incidence of pre-eclampsia, fetal loss, preterm delivery and low birth weight. It is possible to have a satisfactory outcome but careful regular monitoring of blood pressure, renal function and fetal growth is required.

Patients with renal failure sufficient to require haemodialysis have only a very small chance of a normal pregnancy. After successful transplantation pregnancy frequently has a satisfactory outcome. Immunosuppression does not appear to have a harmful effect on the fetus.


## RETROPERITONEAL FIBROSIS

**Introduction.** This is an unusual condition of unknown aetiology which produces an obstructive uropathy due to external compression of the ureters.

**Aetiology**
1. Idiopathic, where no causative agent is found. There may be an autoimmune aetiology as many patients have Raynaud's phenomena and a positive ANF.
2. Drug induced. Methysergide is the most commonly associated but ergotamine, hydralazine and dexamphetamine have all been implicated.

**Pathology.** The ureters are encircled and compressed by dense sclerotic tissue. The tissue arises from the retroperitoneum and is composed of fibrous tissue which may contain inflammatory cells, polymorphs, plasma cells and lymphocytes. The pathogenesis is unknown.

**Clinical Manifestations**
1. It is most common between the ages of 30 and 50.
2. It is more common in males than females.
3. Dull low backache is a common presentation.

4. The patient may complain of polyuria and/or nocturia due to a diabetes insipidus-like syndrome. The urinary back pressure interferes with the renal concentrating ability.
5. Oedema of the legs may be present due to involvement of the inferior vena cava.
6. Rarely the first manifestation may be anuria due to complete ureteric obstruction.

### Investigations and Diagnosis

1. Renal function may be impaired but this is variable.
2. Urinary concentration may be impaired.
3. Proteinuria of up to 1 g daily.
4. The ESR is usually elevated.
5. In some patients the ANF is positive without any signs or other evidence of SLE.
6. Intravenous pyelography may show hydronephrosis and megaureter. The dilated ureter commonly shows tapering towards the pelvic brim and it may also appear to be pulled towards the midline. The lower segment of the ureter fails to fill.
7. Retrograde pyelography reveals similar findings. Usually the catheters pass with ease. Screening will reveal the absence of any peristalsis in the segment of ureter bound by the fibrosis. In many instances one side appears to be more involved than the other.

### Management

1. Establish diagnosis by i.v.p. and retrograde pyelography.
2. Determine the extent of renal impairment.
3. Obtain a full drug history and withdraw any medications which may be causally implicated.
4. Steroids, starting with prednisone 60 mg daily for 4 weeks and thereafter gradually reducing.
5. Regular monitoring of renal function. Isotope renography is of particular value.
6. Surgery to free the ureter from the encasing fibrosis (ureterolysis) should be undertaken: (1) if renal function continues to deteriorate in spite of steroids, (2) if there is evidence of continued obstruction in spite of adequate therapy, and (3) if there is any doubt as to the nature of the fibrosis.

**Prognosis.** This is good in most treated cases, and is to a large part dependent on the degree of renal damage present on diagnosis.


### SICKLE-CELL DISEASE

Patients with sickle-cell disease or trait may have certain renal abnormalities.

**1. Urinary Concentration Defect.** This is probably the earliest manifestation of renal involvement and is found in almost all homozygous patients and many who are heterozygous. The concentrating defect becomes more marked with age. In the early stages the defect is reversible following transfusion with normal red blood cells. It is probably produced by impaired medullary blood supply.

**2. Medullary Infarcts** and **Papillary Necrosis** may occur due to sickling in the medullary blood vessels with subsequent thrombosis and ischaemia. This may rarely be precipitated by flying at high altitudes in unpressurized aircraft.

**3. Haematuria** usually occurs in early adult life and is frequently unilateral and accompanied by colic. The haematuria may be so severe as to require nephrectomy.

**4. Glomerulonephritis** of the subendothelial type of mesangiocapillary glomerulonephritis has been reported. This may produce a nephrotic syndrome.

## BARTTER'S SYNDROME

This is a rare syndrome usually presenting as failure to thrive in early childhood or late infancy. The clinical presentation includes muscle weakness, polyuria, thirst, tetany and constipation. The patients are normotensive.

The biochemical findings are:
1. Hypokalaemic metabolic alkalosis.
2. Elevated plasma renin activity.
3. Increased aldosterone excretion.
4. Renal sodium wasting.

On renal biopsy there is juxtaglomerular cell hyperplasia and prominence of the macula densa.

The pathogenesis of this condition is unknown but it is known that there is increased prostaglandin production. It is postulated that this stimulates renin release from the juxtaglomerular apparatus with subsequent aldosterone production. It is thought that the normotension is due to resistance of blood vessels to the effect of angiotensin II.

Treatment is with either indomethacin or ibuprofen as both inhibit prostaglandin synthetase activity. Therapy, which must be long term, produces a prompt return to biochemical normality and resolution of the clinical features.

## SEGMENTAL HYPOPLASIA (ASK–UPMARK KIDNEY)

Segmental hypoplasia is a rare condition where there is severe segmental renal atrophy frequently associated with hypertension. It is detected most commonly in young adults and there is a female : male ratio of 2 : 1.

The cause of the lesion is not known but initially it was considered to be a congenital lesion as it is rare to find glomerular tissue in the hypoplastic segments. However, recent studies have shown that vesico-ureteric reflux is common and there is a strong association with ureteric abnormalities and renal lithiasis. It is possible therefore that it is a consequence of infection which has gained access by means of vesico-ureteric reflux.

The lesion consists of a localized atrophic scar which appears as a deep groove on intravenous pyelography. The atrophic area involves both cortex and medulla and within this area there are only remnants of normal tissue. Blood vessels are numerous and prominent but this is probably only due to the loss of the intervening parenchyma.

The management consists of:

1.  Controlling the hypertension (*see* Chapter 6).
2.  Maintaining sterile urine.
3.  Repeated assessments of renal growth and function.
4.  Vesico-ureteric reflux with frequent urinary infections may require ureteric reimplantation.
5.  Surgical removal of the hypoplastic segment may be of value if the blood pressure is difficult to control.


## TUMOURS OF THE KIDNEY

Primary tumours of the kidney are not common.

### Malignant Tumours

HYPERNEPHROMA (RENAL CARCINOMA, ADENOCARCINOMA). The term 'hypernephroma' is accepted by common usage but it is incorrect. It was considered originally that the tumour arose from adrenocortical tissue that had become embedded in the kidney during embryonic development. It is now considered that this tumour arises from renal tissue and is not related to the adrenal gland.

Hypernephroma accounts for 80 per cent of renal neoplasms, is most common in the fifth and sixth decades, and has a male preponderance (M : F, 2:1). It occurs equally in the right and left kidney although some cases appear to develop bilaterally. The presenting symptoms are haematuria with a mass and pain in the flank, sometimes the presentation is due to symptoms from metastases. Clinical signs include fever, anaemia and an elevated ESR. In about 5 per cent of patients there is polycythaemia without leucocytosis or thrombocytopenia. The pathogenesis of this is unknown but it has been suggested that the tumour or the surrounding compressed tissue produces erythropoietin. A second laboratory finding of interest is hypercalcaemia which in some cases is due to bony metastases while in other patients is present without any evidence of bony spread. In these cases it is probably due to the secretion of a parathyroid hormone-like substance by the tumour.

The diagnosis of renal carcinoma is made by the finding of a space-occupying lesion on i.v.p. and subsequent investigations showing typical abnormalities. An arteriogram can confirm the space-occupying lesion and demonstrate a typical tumour vascular pattern with, in some cases, the venous phase showing tumour growing along the renal veins. The angiographic demonstration of the tumour circulation can be improved by the infusion of adrenaline which constricts normal arterioles but not the tumour vessels. Ultrasound can differentiate between a tumour and a simple cyst in over 90 per cent of cases.

The hypernephroma is usually irregularly lobulated and may be solitary or multiple. In large tumours necrosis and cyst formation may occur. Calcification frequently occurs. The tumour spreads by (1) local infiltration through the renal capsule, (2) along renal veins, and (3) metastases to bone, lung and brain. The pulmonary lesions may regress after removal of the primary. Bone deposits are osteoclastic.

Management is by:

1. Detailed investigation to demonstrate the size and degree of extension of the tumour.
2. Investigation to determine the presence and extent of metastatic spread.
3. Surgical excision possibly after tumour embolization with Gelfoam.
4. There does not yet appear to be any satisfactory chemotherapy and radiotherapy is not of proven value.

The prognosis is poor with a 35 per cent 5-year survival following nephrectomy in patients with no metastases. Patients with renal vein extensions have a poor prognosis. Metastases may appear many years after removal of the primary.

NEPHROBLASTOMA (WILMS' TUMOUR, EMBRYOMA). This tumour accounts for some 20 per cent of malignancies in childhood. It has a peak incidence at age 3 but it has been demonstrated in neonates and rarely occurs in adolescents and adults. It has a male preponderance (M : F, 2 : 1).

It is usually discovered as a mass in the flank by the child's parents. Less commonly it presents as pain due to local spread.

It is normally solitary, frequently has a rapid growth and is highly malignant. Anaemia is common but haematuria is rare. In early lesions there is a fibrous capsule but in time there is invasion through this to the surrounding tissues such as adrenal, liver, intestines and vertebrae. In addition to local invasion the tumour metastasizes to lungs, liver and brain.

Management is by surgical excision and radiotherapy.

The prognosis is variable and patients treated during the first year of life have the best prognosis. If there are no demonstrable metastases then there is an 80 per cent cure with combined nephrectomy, chemotherapy and radiotherapy. If the patient survives two years from nephrectomy then the overall outlook is good.

### Benign Tumours

HAEMANGIOPERICYTOMA. This is a rare tumour which has no age or sex predilection. It is a well-demarcated tumour which grows slowly. It is richly vascular and is thought to arise from perivascular tissue. It may secrete renin and therefore produce hypertension. Diagnosis is by demonstrating renin-mediated hypertension (*see* Chapter 6) and localization can be achieved by selective renal venous sampling. Renal arteriography usually reveals a small vascular lesion. Management is by control of hypertension and surgical excision.

ANGIOMYOLIPOMATA. These are small, frequently multiple and bilateral cortical tumours consisting of fat cells, fibrous tissue, smooth muscle and atypical blood vessels. They are found in association with tuberous sclerosis. They produce no functional impairment and are of little clinical significance.

# Chapter 15

# DRUGS AND THE KIDNEY

Diuretic therapy – Drug therapy in impaired renal function – Dialysis of drugs – Drug nephrotoxicity

## DIURETIC THERAPY

**Introduction.** Diuretics are drugs which act on the kidney and promote an increased rate of urine flow. The major indications for the use of these drugs are:
1. Elimination of excess sodium in oedematous states such as in the nephrotic syndrome, congestive cardiac failure or cirrhosis.
2. As an adjunct in the management of hypertension.
3. In severe chronic renal failure in an attempt to increase urine volume and thus allow a more liberal fluid intake.
4. In the early phase of acute renal failure in an attempt to maintain an adequate urine flow.
5. To increase greatly the rate of turnover of extracellular fluid in intoxication states.

**Site of Action.** Diuretics can act at various sites in the nephron. Sometimes it is necessary to use a combination of diuretic drugs and in such situations it is necessary to prescribe preparations which act at different sites. For instance in severe nephrotic syndrome there is maximal salt and water retention and 'loop' diuretics, although acting at the thick ascending limb of the loop of Henle, may not produce a diuresis because of distal reabsorption due to secondary aldosteronism. Similarly the blocking of the action of aldosterone alone may be ineffective as little sodium may be delivered to the late part of the distal tubule. In such states it is reasonable to combine frusemide or ethacrynic acid with spironolactone.
1. AFFERENT ARTERIOLE: Aminophylline; Digoxin
   Drugs which cause an increased renal perfusion, and thereby an increase in glomerular filtration, frequently promote a diuresis. The mechanism of action is probably by the abolition of intrarenal compensatory mechanisms induced by poor renal perfusion.
   An increase in renal blood flow has been demonstrated following frusemide administration.
2. PROXIMAL TUBULE
   *Osmotic Agents:* Mannitol; Glucose
   Non-resorbable substances which increase the osmotic pressure of the intratubular fluid diminish iso-osmotic absorption.
   *Carbonic Anhydrase Inhibitors:* Acetazolamide
   Bicarbonate reabsorption may be impaired by carbonic anhydrase inhibitors and the increased tubular bicarbonate acts as a

non-reabsorbable anion which induces an osmotic diuresis. The effect is self-limiting as once the plasma bicarbonate concentration falls the filtered load of bicarbonate falls and therefore its osmotic effect is less.

*Frusemide* in a high dose (> 500 mg) has a proximal tubular effect.

3. THICK ASCENDING LIMB OF THE LOOP OF HENLE: Frusemide; Bumetanide; Ethacrynic acid

In the thick ascending limb of the loop of Henle active chloride transport associated with a passive sodium flux occurs. The so-called 'loop' diuretics block chloride reabsorption and are the most potent diuretics available. These drugs also act on the first part of the distal tubule.

4. DISTAL TUBULE: Thiazides; Metolazone; Chlorthalidone

Sodium reabsorption in the distal tubule can be blocked thereby producing a diuresis.

5. LATE DISTAL TUBULE

*Blocking of Sodium Reabsorption*: Amiloride; Triamterene

The blockage of sodium reabsorption from the lumen at this site effectively inhibits the action of aldosterone.

*Competitive Inhibition of Aldosterone*: Spironolactone

In the late distal tubule sodium/potassium exchange takes place under the influence of aldosterone and thus any inhibition of aldosterone promotes a natriuresis.

*Note*: Diuretics acting at this site do not require the addition of potassium supplements.

6. INHIBITION OF THE ACTION OF VASOPRESSIN: Lithium; Demethylchlortetracycline; Chlorpropamide; Alcohol

The action of vasopressin can be blocked and thus the formation of a concentrated urine can be inhibited. These drugs are not used as diuretics but have an important role in conditions of excessive or inappropriate ADH secretion.

**Dosage of Individual Drugs.** The choice of a diuretic will depend to a large extent on the clinical situation. In hypertension and mild cardiac failure those acting on the distal tubule are most appropriate. In emergency situations or severe oedematous states the 'loop' diuretics, possibly combined with later acting preparations, are best. In resistant cases high doses may be necessary but care should be taken to determine the cause of the so-called 'resistance' and toxicity must be avoided.

MANNITOL. Normal adult dosage is 200 ml of 20 per cent solution i.v. Care must be taken to prevent cardiac failure.

AMINOPHYLLINE. 250 mg i.v. or 360 mg suppositories.

ACETAZOLAMIDE (Diamox). 250–500 mg daily. The best effect is obtained by an alternate-day regimen.

FRUSEMIDE (Lasix). 40 mg tablets. There is a wide therapeutic range but normally 20–80 mg daily is adequate. In refractory oedema or severe renal failure dosages of 500–1000 mg may be used (500 mg tablets are available). A parenteral preparation is available.

BUMETANIDE (Burinex). 1 mg tablets. The diuretic response of bumetanide is similar to that of 40–60 mg frusemide. Parenteral preparation available.

ETHACRYNIC ACID (Edecrin). 50 mg tablets. Dosage normally 50–100 mg daily. Parenteral preparation available.

THIAZIDES. There is no good evidence that one thiazide is clinically more effective than another.

*Bendrofluazide* (Aprinox, Neo-Naclex): 5–10 mg daily.

*Hydrochlorothiazide* (Hydrosaluric): 50–200 mg daily.

*Polythiazide* (Nephril): 1–4 mg daily.

METOLAZONE (Zaroxolyn). 5–20 mg daily.

CHLORTHALIDONE (Hygroton). 50–200 mg daily. The site of action is the same as for thiazides although the duration of action is more prolonged.

AMILORIDE (Midamor). 5–20 mg daily.

TRIAMTERENE (Dytac). 150–250 mg daily.

SPIRONOLACTONE (Aldactone). 100–400 mg daily.

**Side Effects**

1. Potassium depletion: probably the most recognized complication but seldom producing problems. Must be carefully avoided especially if the patient is also receiving digoxin. In any patient if the plasma potassium falls below 3·5 mmol/l potassium chloride supplements are indicated. Late distal tubule-acting diuretics do not need potassium supplements.

2. Volume depletion: this may be severe, particularly if hypovolaemia was present prior to commencing therapy. May produce postural hypotension.

3. Hyponatraemia: may develop due to impaired free water excretion.

4. Hyperuricaemia: particularly with thiazides and 'loop' diuretics.

5. Hypersensitivity reactions: dermatitis, pneumonitis, vasculitis, purpura and interstitial nephritis.

6. Cramp.

7. Deafness: particularly with intravenous high dose frusemide, especially in impaired renal function.

8. Gastrointestinal upset.

9. Abnormal glucose tolerance, particularly with frusemide and thiazides.

**Idiopathic Oedema and Diuretics.** Idiopathic oedema is a term used to describe oedema of unknown cause and mainly found in young women. These patients are frequently associated with the medical profession. They regularly take diuretics but it is often unclear why they commenced their treatment. On stopping the drugs they develop increase in weight and oedema probably due to the physiological responses evoked by prolonged diuretic-induced hypovolaemia. If, however, the patient can be persuaded to desist from further diuretic therapy this oedema and weight gain resolves.

## DRUG THERAPY IN IMPAIRED RENAL FUNCTION

**Introduction.** Many drugs and their metabolites are excreted by the kidney and therefore it is often necessary to alter drug regimen in patients with renal failure. Unmodified dosage leads to:
1. High plasma concentrations.
2. Prolonged activity.
3. An increased incidence of side effects.

Patients with renal failure usually require a normal initial drug dosage schedule to achieve adequate therapeutic plasma concentrations. This should then be followed by a prolongation of the time intervals between doses and/or reduction in dosage to achieve an effective drug concentration. To ensure that adequate therapy is being maintained it is necessary in many instances to monitor plasma concentrations, and it is best to determine the 'peak' value (usually 1 hour after adminstration) and the 'trough' value (immediately prior to next dose). Caution must be exercised in uraemia and the nephrotic syndrome where low plasma protein binding may be associated with a relatively high 'free' drug concentration although the total plasma concentration may appear acceptable. A similar situation may arise in severe acidosis.

**Antibiotics**

ANTITUBERCULOUS DRUGS. Isoniazid and rifampicin are excreted mainly by the liver and no alteration in dosage is required. Ethambutol, if used, should be given on an alternate-day regimen while PAS should be avoided.

AMINOGLYCOSIDES (gentamicin, tobramycin, kanamycin). These drugs are nephrotoxic and ototoxic and must be used with extreme caution in renal failure. Normal loading doses are required and monitoring of plasma concentrations are required during therapy. Plasma concentrations in excess of 8 $\mu$g/ml for gentamicin and tobramycin are to be avoided.

CEPHALOSPORINS. This group may be nephrotoxic, particularly in high dosage and when combined with aminoglycosides, diuretics or in the presence of hypovolaemia. If a cephalosporin is indicated then cephradine (Velocef) should be used.

CLINDAMYCIN. Dosage unchanged but the risk of pseudomembranous colitis exists.

ERYTHROMYCIN. Excreted by the liver, dosage unchanged in renal failure.

LINCOMYCIN. Mainly excreted by liver but dose must be reduced in severe renal failure.

NALIDIXIC ACID. Mainly excreted by liver but metabolites may accumulate as they are excreted by the kidney.

NITROFURANTOIN. Accumulation of metabolites may produce a peripheral sensory neuropathy and thus its use in severe renal failure should be avoided.

PENICILLINS. Fairly safe but may cause interstitial nephritis (particularly methicillin). High plasma concentrations may produce encephalopathy. Many penicillins are prepared as the sodium or potassium salt and if high dosage (such as with carbenicillin) is used this may produce unexpected electrolyte disorders.

SULPHONAMIDES. Excreted by the kidney and dosage must be reduced in severe renal failure. Early drugs in this group, such as sulphadiazine, sometimes produced acute obstructive uropathy due to intratubular crystal deposition.

TETRACYCLINES. Doxycycline and minocycline are the only members of this group which may be used in renal failure. Others must be avoided as they potentiate acidosis and raise plasma urea. In severe chronic renal failure they may produce an acute and often irreversible deterioration in renal function.

VANCOMYCIN. Monitoring of plasma concentration essential in renal failure.

### Analgesics

ASPIRIN. Side effects such as gastrointestinal bleeding more prominent. Protein binding reduced in severe renal failure therefore dosage must be reduced.

PARACETAMOL. Excreted mainly by the liver. Use with caution in severe renal failure. Distalgesic (dextropropoxyphene 32·5 mg plus paracetamol 325 mg) is a useful analgesic in renal failure.

MORPHINE. Excreted by the liver and can be used in normal dosage.

### Hypnotics and Tranquillizers

BENZODIAZEPINES. Most members of this group are excreted by the liver and can be used in normal dosage. In some patients excessive sedation may occur and dosage has to be reduced. Severe neurological sequelae have been observed in dialysis patients and thus cautious use is advised.

HALOPERIDOL. Normal dosage.

PHENOTHIAZINES. May cause urinary retention but normally no change in dosage regimen required.

TRICYCLIC ANTIDEPRESSANTS. Most can be used in unchanged dosage. May decrease the hypotensive effect of bethanidine, guanethidine and debrisoquine.

### Cardiovascular Drugs

DIGOXIN. Normal loading dose required but maintenance therapy reduced. Plasma concentrations and careful enquiry regarding toxicity essential. Hypokalaemia potentiates toxicity.

HYPOTENSIVE AGENTS. Blood pressure response is best guide to dosage and frequency. In renal failure there is a theoretical advantage in using agents which cause vasodilatation such as hydralazine and prazosin. Methyldopa remains a valuable agent although side effects more common. Beta-blockers are of value although care must be used in severe failure.

### Miscellaneous Drugs

IMMUNOSUPPRESSIVE AGENTS. Should be used with caution as their action may be prolonged.

CLOFIBRATE. In nephrotic syndrome side effects potentiated.

ANTACIDS. Aluminium-containing compounds may have an adverse effect on bone metabolism and may, in dialysis patients, be responsible for encephalopathy. Magnesium-containing compounds may produce hypermagnesaemia.

## DIALYSIS OF DRUGS

Haemodialysis and peritoneal dialysis are capable of removing drugs from the circulation. Generally drugs which are water soluble and poorly bound to proteins are capable of elimination by haemodialysis. Peritoneal dialysis is relatively inefficient in drug removal due to low clearance rates.

Dialysis may be associated with:

1. Removal of drug in an overdose situation. There are few drugs which fall into this category and it may well be that the charcoal haemoperfusion proves to be more efficient.
2. Removal of a drug which is required therapeutically. This may require the giving of an additional dose during dialysis, e.g. a patient on anticonvulsant therapy may have the concentration of a drug reduced by dialysis and therefore be liable to have a fit. This can be overcome by alteration of drug regimen.
3. Electrolyte changes, such as a reduction in plasma potassium, may potentiate digoxin toxicity.

## DRUG NEPHROTOXICITY

**Introduction.** Drug-induced renal disease is of importance inasmuch as it is avoidable in many cases. It is essential to be aware of certain associations as patients requiring potentially nephrotoxic drugs can be monitored in an attempt to detect toxicity early. In many instances it is the abuse of a drug which has led to renal damage.

A wide variety of syndromes can be produced by drugs.

**Interstitial Nephritis**
1. ACUTE. This may develop some 7–14 days after intitial exposure and patients frequently have fever, eosinophilia and skin rash. Methicillin, frusemide, thiazides, rifampicin and sulphonamides have been implicated.
2. CHRONIC. Analgesic abuse is the most common cause. As many analgesic preparations are compound tablets it is difficult to be certain which agent is responsible but phenacetin is most likely. Most patients will deny abuse.

**Acute Tubular Necrosis.** Many drugs are capable of producing acute tubular necrosis but a causal effect is often difficult to establish due to the complex clinical situations which are usually present. Aminoglycosides (particularly when combined with diuretics), cephalosporins, tetracycline, carbon tetrachloride and sulphonamides have all been implicated. Management is by withdrawal of the drug and supportive measures including dialysis until renal function recovers. In patients with chronic renal failure acute deterioration in renal function may follow hypovolaemia induced by vomiting and/or diarrhoea. Many drugs may produce gastrointestinal upset and this again emphasizes the care which must be taken when prescribing for patients with poor renal function.

**Tubular Damage** (not amounting to necrosis). Intravenous amphotericin produces distal tubular damage which can be reversible or permanent.

**Obstructive Nephropathy**
1. INTRARENAL. This may result from drug crystal deposition as in therapy with some sulphonamides, or uric acid crystal formation following massive cellular destruction during chemotherapy for leukaemia.
2. EXTRARENAL. Ureteric obstruction from retroperitoneal fibrosis has been associated with methysergide and rarely following therapy with ergotamine, hydralazine and methyldopa.

**Nephrotic Syndrome.** This may occur during therapy with gold, penicillamine, mercurial compounds, anticonvulsants, levamisole, tolbutamide and in heroin abuse. The lesion produced is frequently a membranous glomerulonephritis which in most instances resolves following withdrawal of the drug concerned.

**Acute Vasculitis.** This is rare but has been reported following penicillin, sulphonamide or thiazide therapy. The lesions produced are similar to those found in polyarteritis nodosa.

**Drug-induced Lupus Erythematosus.** A syndrome similar to spontaneous systemic lupus erythematosus has been described following therapy with hydralazine, isoniazid and procainamide. Renal involvement occurs much less than in the spontaneous form and usually resolves following withdrawal of the drug.

**Analgesic Nephropathy.** Excessive analgesic consumption is a well-recognized and important cause of chronic renal failure. Phenacetin was considered to be the drug responsible for producing the renal lesion but now it is considered that other agents, such as codeine, aspirin and paracetamol may be important.

The underlying lesion is vascular damage leading to papillary necrosis with secondary atrophy of the involved nephrons. The clinical features are polyuria and polydipsia due to impairment of the renal concentrating ability. Renal colic and haematuria may result from sloughing of necrotic papillae. Diagnosis is frequently difficult as patients are reluctant to admit to excessive analgesic consumption and although the i.v.p. may show characteristic changes it may be surprisingly normal. Management is by abolishing, if possible, analgesic intake.